8/06
B+T
11.00

W9-AAE-003

SEP 0 4 2006
MAR 1 6 2007

WALNUT PUBLIC LIBRARY DIST.
Heaton & Main St. Box 728
WALNUT, IL 61376-0728

healthy
weight loss

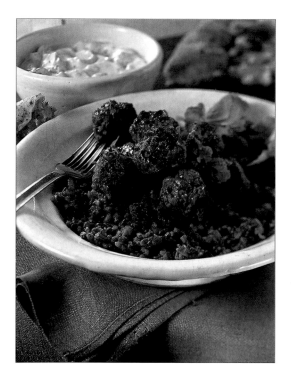

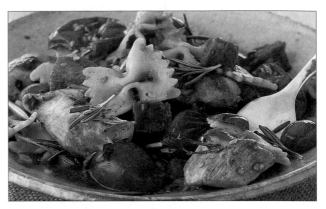

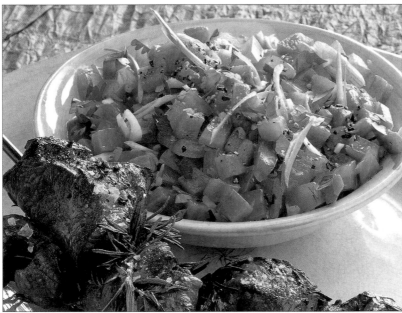

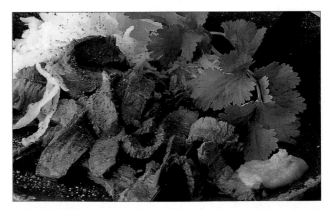

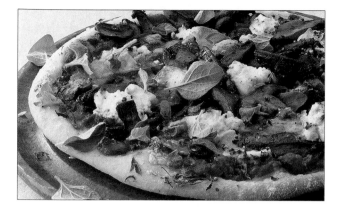

healthy
weight loss

ESSENTIAL ADVICE ON HOW TO LOSE WEIGHT WITHOUT
MISSING OUT ON DELICIOUS, APPETIZING MEALS

CONTRIBUTING EDITOR: FIONA HUNTER

LORENZ BOOKS

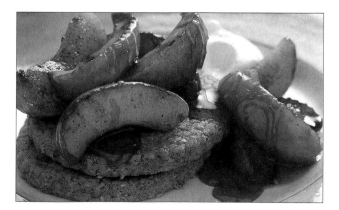

This edition is published by Lorenz Books

Lorenz Books is an imprint of Anness Publishing Ltd
Hermes House, 88–89 Blackfriars Road, London SE1 8HA
tel. 020 7401 2077; fax 020 7633 9499; www.lorenzbooks.com; info@anness.com

© Anness Publishing Ltd 2000, 2003

This edition distributed in the UK by Aurum Press Ltd, 25 Bedford Avenue, London WC1B 3AT
tel. 020 7637 3225; fax 020 7580 2469

This edition distributed in the USA and Canada by National Book Network, 4720 Boston Way, Lanham, MD 20706
tel. 301 459 3366; fax 301 459 1705; www.nbnbooks.com

This edition distributed in Australia by Pan Macmillan Australia, Level 18, St Martins Tower, 31 Market St
Sydney, NSW 2000; tel. 1300 135 113; fax 1300 135 103; customer.service@macmillan.com.au

This edition distributed in New Zealand by David Bateman Ltd, 30 Tarndale Grove, Off Bush Road
Albany, Auckland; tel. (09) 415 7664; fax (09) 415 8892

All rights reserved. No part of this publication may be reproduced, stored in a retrieval system, or transmitted in
any way or by any means, electronic, mechanical, photocopying, recording or otherwise, without the prior written
permission of the copyright holder.

A CIP catalogue record for this book is available from the British Library

Publisher: Joanna Lorenz
Executive Editor: Linda Fraser
Editor: Finny Fox-Davies
Designer: Julie Francis
Illustrations: Lucinda Ganderton
Reader: Jan Cutler
Production Controller: Lee Sargent
Photographers: Edward Allwright, James Duncan, Gus Filgate, Michelle Garrett, Amanda Heywood, Fiona Hunter,
Dave Jordan, Dave King, William Lingwood, Thomas Odulate, David Reilly and Sam Stowell
(Pictures on pp 7, 8 and 9 were supplied by Tony Stone Images)
Recipes: Trish Davies, Matthew Drennan, Joanna Farrow, Silvana Franco, Shirley Gill, Nicola Graimes, Carole
Handslip, Christine Ingram, Manisha Kanahi, Sue Maggs, Sally Mansfield, Liz Trigg, Steven Wheeler and Jeni Wright

Also published as *The Weight-Loss Cookbook*

1 3 5 7 9 10 8 6 4 2

NOTES
For all recipes, quantities are given in both metric and imperial measures
and, where appropriate, measures are also given in standard cups and
spoons. Follow one set, but not a mixture, because they are not
interchangeable.

Standard spoon and cup measures are level.
1 tsp = 5ml, 1 tbsp = 15ml, 1 cup = 250ml/8fl oz

Australian standard tablespoons are 20ml. Australian readers should
use 3 tsp in place of 1 tbsp for measuring small quantities of gelatine,
cornflour, salt, etc.

Medium (US large) eggs are used unless otherwise stated.

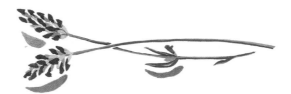

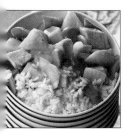

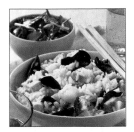

CONTENTS

Introduction 6
The Energy Balance Equation 8
Choosing the Right Diet 10
Getting Started 12
Slimline Shopping 14
Cooking Light 18
Trimming the Fat 19
Counting the Calories 20
Putting it All into Practice 24

Breakfast 26

Starters and Light Meals 36

Meat, Poultry and Seafood 52

Vegetables, Grains and Pulses 68

Desserts 84

Index 96

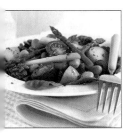

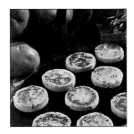

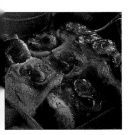

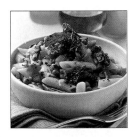

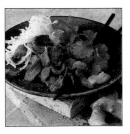

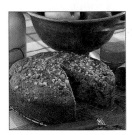

INTRODUCTION

There is no doubt that the food we eat can have an important effect on our health and well-being. A healthy diet can help us live longer and remain healthier throughout our lives; help protect against heart disease, cancer, diabetes and obesity; increase our resistance to colds and other infections; boost energy levels and help us cope better with the stresses of modern living.

The good news is that choosing a healthy diet doesn't mean that you are condemned to a life of eating mung beans, brown rice and cottage cheese, nor does it have to mean saying goodbye to the foods you enjoy. Small changes in the foods you choose and the way you prepare them can make a big difference and can be a positive step towards better health.

A BALANCED APPROACH

The secret to a healthy diet lies in balance, moderation and variety. There are no such things as "good" and "bad" or "healthy" and "unhealthy" foods; it's what you eat most of the time that matters. Even small changes, like switching from full-fat to skimmed or semi-skimmed milk, or from white to wholemeal bread, can make a significant difference. Eating a wide variety of foods is important to ensure that your diet provides the full range of nutrients necessary for good health. The key to successful weight control is knowing what foods to eat and in what quantities to eat them. Some foods, particularly those that are high in fat, contain lots of calories, but this doesn't mean that you need to avoid them completely, simply that you need to be careful with the amount you eat. Other foods, such as fruit, vegetables, lean meat, fish and chicken, are lower in calories and can be eaten in more generous quantities.

THE IDEAL BODY WEIGHT

Losing weight isn't easy, but the benefits are enormous – you'll feel fitter and more confident, you'll have more energy and you'll be healthier. Being overweight increases the risk of a number of serious health problems, in particular diabetes, heart disease, high blood pressure, stroke, reproductive disorders, gallstones, osteoarthritis and certain types of cancer. In the past, ideal weight has been determined using charts, which give the ideal weight for men and women of different heights and builds. This method of determining ideal body weight has fallen out of favour nowadays and has been replaced by a measurement known as Body Mass Index or BMI.

Your body composition – how much of your weight is fat and where that fat is stored in the body – is another important factor in determining the health risks associated

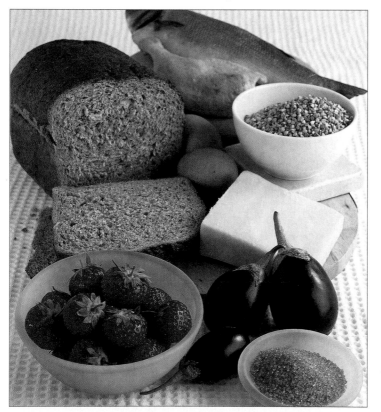

Left: In a balanced diet, nothing is forbidden, though some foods should have a higher profile than others. Eat plenty of fruit, vegetables, lean meat, fish and chicken, for example.

with being overweight. Measuring the waist to hip ratio is often used as a guide to the distribution of fat around the body. In order to calculate this, divide your waist measurement by your hip measurement: if the ratio is greater than 0.85 for women and greater than 0.95 for men, you're carrying too much fat around your waist.

In fact, however, it is no longer really necessary to do the number crunching, since experts now believe that a measure of waist circumference alone is a pretty good measure of both central fat and total fatness. A waist circumference of over 102cm/40in for men and over 88cm/35in for women suggests that there is a serious need to lose weight.

HOW YOU SHAPE UP

Apples and pears: Fat that is stored around the waist, producing an apple-shaped body, is more likely to be linked with health problems, particularly an increased risk of non-insulin diabetes, heart disease, high blood pressure and abnormal blood fat levels. In women, central obesity is associated with a higher risk of premenopausal breast cancer. Fat that is stored around the hips in what is generally described as a pear shape, seems to be rather less problematic.

The reason why the apple distribution of fat should be more harmful to health than the pear distribution is not clearly understood. One theory is that central fat is more metabolically active and causes changes in the levels of blood fats, which increase the risk of heart disease.

Whether you're an "apple" or a "pear" is partly inherited. However, certain factors such as smoking and alcohol seem to increase the likelihood for fat to be laid down in the stomach area, while exercise helps reduce stomach fat. The good news is that there is some evidence to suggest that it is easier to lose central fat than that stored around the hips.

HOW YOU SHAPE UP

There is no exact correct weight for good health. Instead there is a healthy weight range and you should aim for a weight somewhere within this. The Body Mass Index is the most valid indication of weight status, and studies have shown that men and women from 18 years onwards with a BMI between 20 and 25 have the least risk of disease and death. If you have a small frame, you should aim for the lower end of the healthy weight range, if you are large-framed or exercise a lot, look to higher levels.

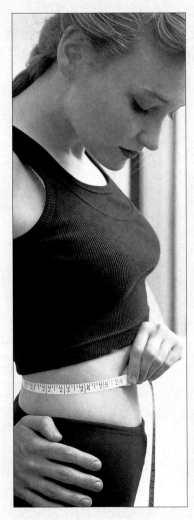

• **Body Mass Index (BMI):** This index measures fat levels by plotting your weight (in kilograms) versus your height (in meters) squared. This index gives a measure of what is underweight, healthy and overweight by height.

For example 60kg ÷ (1.65m x 1.65m) = 22

• For men and women from 18 years onwards:
Below 18.5   =   underweight
18.5-25   =   acceptable
25-30   =   overweight
30-40   =   obese
Over 40   =   severely obese

To convert units:
2.2lb = 1kg
39.37in = 1m

• **Waist circumference as a means of determining fat levels:** A quick and easy indication is to be found by measuring your waist. You need to lose weight if your waist measures:
over 102cm/40in in men
over 88cm/35in in women

Left: Measuring your waist will give you a fairly accurate measure of both central fat and total fatness, and an indication of whether you need to lose weight or not.

THE ENERGY BALANCE EQUATION

There is no mystery as to why we gain weight – it's a simple equation. We gain weight when the energy (calories) we consume exceeds the energy we use. In this situation, excess energy is stored on the body as fat. Eating just a small amount in excess of your needs will result in a slow but steady weight gain. Thus eating just 100 calories a day more than you need – the equivalent of 1½ digestive biscuits – will result in a weight gain of 4.7kg/10lb in a year. To lose weight, you simply need to tip the balance so you use more calories than you consume, and the body will draw on fat reserves to provide the energy it needs. You can do this by restricting the number of calories you eat or by increasing the amount of calories you use, but without doubt the best way is a combination of diet and exercise.

COUNTING THE CALORIES

The basis of any weight-reducing diet is to bring down the number of calories you consume. But what exactly is a calorie? It's the unit used to measure the energy value of food and also the energy requirements of the body. The scientific definition of one calorie is the amount of heat required to raise the temperature of 1 gram of water by 1 degree centigrade. The general term used is calories or kilocalories (abbreviated to kcals, or Cals). Energy values can also be measured in kilojoules (kJ), which is the metric equivalent. 1kcal equals 4.2kJ, so to convert kcal to kJ you need to multiply by 4.2.

Energy requirements: Depending on a person's age, sex, level of activity and weight, their energy requirements can vary considerably. The average daily energy requirement for women aged between 19 and 49 years is 1,940 calories. For men between 19 and 49 years, it is 2,550 calories per day. It isn't healthy to reduce your calorie

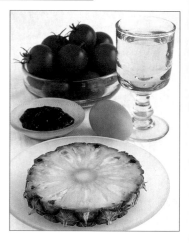

intake too severely in an effort to lose weight. Studies suggest that reducing your calorie intake by 600 calories a day should be enough to produce a weight loss of up to 1kg (2lb) a week, which is ideal. Most women will lose weight on around 1,200–1,500 calories a day (1,500–1,750 calories a day for men). Diets containing fewer than 1,000 calories a day are not recommended without medical supervision because they could lead to loss of lean muscle tissue as well as fat.

Above: Each of the above contains just 100 calories – 450g/1lb tomatoes, .120g/4½oz slice of pineapple, 15ml/1 tbsp jam, 1 egg, 150ml/5fl oz glass of wine.

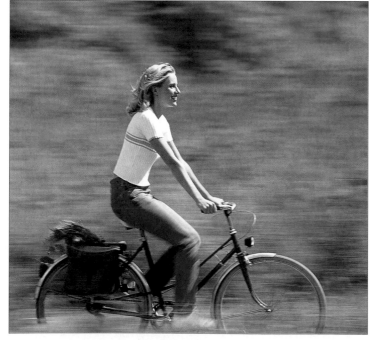

Left: Cycling is an excellent form of exercise, particularly if it is kept up on a regular basis. It can be done at any age, and for short or long periods of time.

THE ROLE OF EXERCISE

If you've ever watched the calories slowly clocking up despite furiously pedalling away on the exercise bike, you will know that on its own, exercise is not a very efficient way of burning calories. But exercise does play an important role in dieting. If you exercise at the same time as dieting, more of the weight you lose will be fat rather than lean muscle tissue. Exercise preserves and develops muscle tissue which is metabolically more active than fat (it uses more calories than fat); so, in other words, the more muscle you have, the more calories your body burns. Exercise can also help to improve your body shape and tone. You don't need to be running a marathon twice a week to reap the benefits of exercise – small changes in routine, such as walking part of the way to work or running up the stairs rather than taking the lift, all increase energy expenditure. The secret is to build exercise into your daily routine, find something that you enjoy which fits in with your lifestyle; be realistic, start slowly and gradually build up the frequency and length of time for which you exercise.

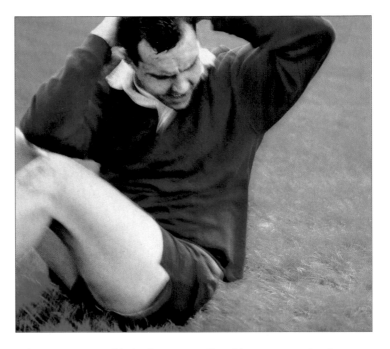

Below: Exercise is one of the key features of controlling energy output. Exercise helps build up more muscles, which are metabolically more active than fat, and improves body shape and tone.

Above: The more you exercise, the more energy you burn up. Most men have larger frames than women, and this means they have more muscle and use more calories than women.

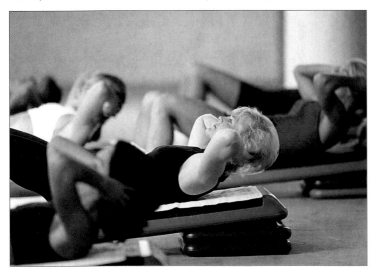

THE INACTIVE SOCIETY

Many nutritionists believe that the real reason for the alarming rise in levels of obesity that we've witnessed over the last decade is not because we're eating more but because we are doing less. An increasing amount of our free time is spent watching television or videos, playing computer games or surfing the Net. Modern technology and labour-saving devices mean that we're much less active than we used to be. The average amount of time spent watching television has doubled to 27 hours a week in just 30 years.

Choosing the Right Diet

Before you embark upon any diet, ask yourself exactly why you're doing it and what you expect to achieve from it. It's always helpful to start by making a list of all the reasons why you want to lose weight. The next step is to decide what your target weight will be. Ensure that you set yourself realistic goals, and if you have a lot of weight to lose it's a good idea to set yourself a series of targets. Then treat yourself to a small reward each time that you reach one of your targets.

When it comes to losing weight, there are no miracle cures. Don't think about dieting as a short-term solution – the only way to lose weight safely and permanently is to make long-term changes in your eating habits and lifestyle. Forget about dieting – think about a whole new way of eating. This doesn't mean banning all your favourite foods – in fact, it's important to include the foods you enjoy. A diet that leaves you feeling deprived and unhappy is a diet that's soon going to be abandoned.

The Facts About Fat

The most effective way of reducing your calorie intake is to keep the amount of fat you eat to a minimum. Foods like butter, oil, cream and fatty meats obviously contain a lot of fat – you can tell just by looking at them. But many other foods also contain fat – biscuits, crisps, ready-made meals and many processed foods often contain large amounts of fat, much of which is hidden. Even reduced-fat foods can contain significant amounts of fat. For example a small packet of reduced-fat crisps still contains 6g fat.

Whatever the type, fat always equals calories, so it is best to keep your intake as low as possible.

High-fat Foods

These include foods such as butter, cream, oil, fatty cuts of meat and processed meats such as sausages and burgers, avocado pears, nuts, oily fish, cheese, creamy sauces, pastry, salad dressing, crisps, snacks, pâté, chocolate, ice cream, some yogurts.

Low-fat diets: Because fat contains twice as many calories as either protein or carbohydrate, low-fat diets are a very effective way of reducing calories. Fat adds flavour and texture to foods,

however, so very low-fat diets can be somewhat bland and unexciting.

Calorie-controlled ready-made meals: These can be useful to keep in the freezer for times when you don't feel like cooking but on the whole you'd be better off making your own.

High-fibre diets: High-fibre foods are filling; they will help you feel full quicker and stop you feeling hungry.

Meal replacement drinks or bars: These are fine occasionally when you don't feel like cooking, but real food always tastes much better.

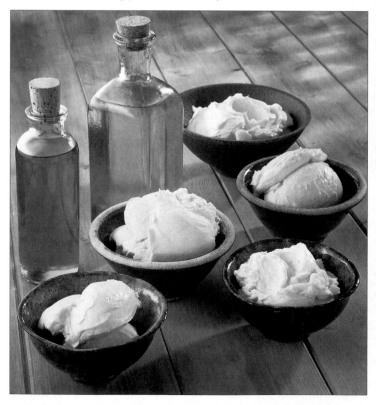

Right: Oils, margarine and butter have the same high calorie count – 145 calories per 15ml/1tbsp. Low-fat spreads and margarines contain about half this level.

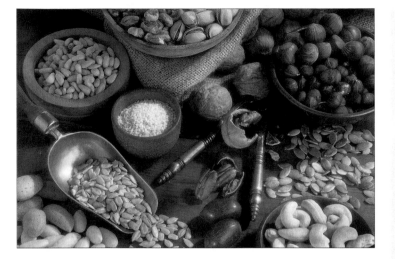

ALL CALORIES ARE NOT EQUAL

If you're following a 1,500-calorie diet, does it really matter whether those calories come from fat, carbohydrate, protein or alcohol?

Where your calories come from can influence how full you feel after eating. Experiments in which volunteers were fed on meals containing an identical number of calories but from different sources clearly demonstrated that meals containing high levels of protein or carbohydrate were more effective at preventing hunger later in the day. High-fat meals did not have the same capacity to hold hunger in check.

THE GLYCEMIC INDEX (GI)

This index measures the rate at which carbohydrate foods are digested and converted into sugar, producing a rise in blood sugar levels. Pure glucose has a GI rating of 100 and is quickly absorbed into the bloodstream. Foods with a low GI rating are broken down more slowly than other foods and will help you feel full for longer.

Right: Beans and other pulses, apples, whole-grain cereals, dried apricots, pasta and oats are all low-GI foods.

Above: Nuts and seeds are very nutritious and rich in dietary fibre, vitamins and minerals. They are also high in fat, though some nuts, such as almonds and walnuts, have good fats. All nuts are high in calories.

DIETS TO AVOID

Crash diets: However tempting they may sound, crash diets are never the answer. Although you may lose weight initially, the chances are you'll end up putting it all back on. They don't teach you how to change your eating habits on a long-term basis, which is essential to keeping weight off.
Food combining diets: Any eating plan that restricts the amount and type of food you can eat will result in weight loss. There's no scientific reason why food combining should work any better than other diet.
Fad diets: The Cabbage Soup Diet, The Beverly Hills Diet – these provide only a short-term fix for a problem that really needs a long-term solution.

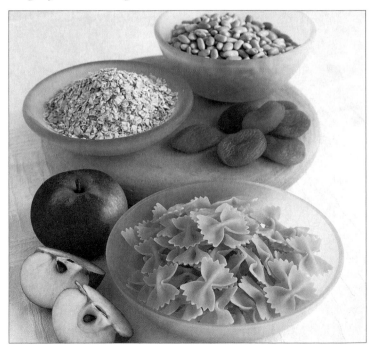

GETTING STARTED

How often have you been tempted by the promise of losing 3kg/7lb in 7 days, only to find that the very next week you've regained all the weight you lost plus a little more? Yo-yo dieting – repeatedly losing and regaining weight – is not regarded as healthy. The best and safest way to lose weight is slowly and steadily – between 1–2lb/ 0.5–1kg a week is thought to be the ideal rate. If, however, you lose too much weight too quickly, there is always a danger that you may lose lean muscle tissue as well as fat. Since the metabolic rate is related to the amount of lean muscle tissue in the body, it's a particularly good idea to do whatever we can to preserve it.

KEEPING A FOOD DIARY

We eat for many different reasons – often it's out of habit rather than hunger. Certain people, places and situations prompt us to eat more than we really should or want to. Keeping a food diary for a couple of weeks will help you identify places, people and moods that cause you to eat more than you intend. Once you have identified these factors, you can work on developing strategies that will help you avoid them. Try keeping a record of everything you eat or drink – buy a notebook and divide the pages into columns as shown below. Write down everything you eat and drink for two weeks and then look back to identify situations where your diet goes astray.

GENERAL GUIDELINES

• Eat three meals a day and don't be tempted to skip any. Eating little and often will help keep blood sugar levels stable and will help you resist the temptation to snack.
• Eat proper meals. Snacking or grazing between meals makes it hard to assess exactly how much you have eaten and makes it more difficult to eat a balanced diet.
• Drink plenty of water; between 6–8 glasses per day/1.75 litres/3 pints is recommended. Drink a glass of water before each meal.
• Be prepared. Make sure that your storecupboard is full of healthy foods, and have a selection of low-calorie snacks available.

• Always remember the 15-minute rule – which is that it takes 15 minutes for your brain to register that your stomach is full. If you still feel hungry at the end of your meal, wait for 15 minutes before you give in and eat anything else. The chances are that, after 15 minutes, you won't feel the need to eat anything else.
• Don't feel that one bad day will ruin the entire diet – it won't. Life is full of ups and downs – so, if you've had a bad day, be extra strict with yourself the next day. Nobody should have to stick to a strict diet on high days and holidays. Instead, if you know you've got a special event coming up soon, be extra careful for a couple of days or so beforehand.

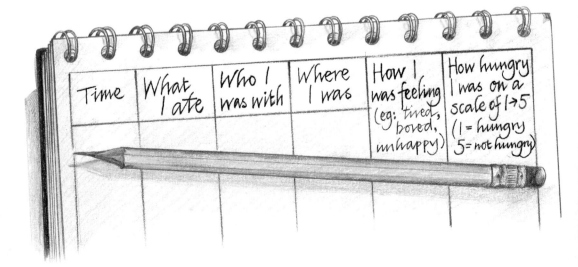

• Never go shopping on an empty stomach. Write a list and stick to it. Don't be tempted to buy crisps or biscuits if you know you won't be able to resist them when you get home.

• Listen to your body – are you really hungry or are you bored, cold or tired? It's easy to confuse feeling thirsty with feeling hungry.

• Don't skip meals. Allowing yourself to get hungry means that when you do eat, you're more likely to overeat.

• High-fibre foods will help you feel full more quickly and keep you from feeling hungry for longer.

• Focus on your food – give food your full attention. If you eat while watching television or reading, you are more likely to miss signals saying you are full.

• Eat slowly and chew your food thoroughly – remember the brain takes 15 minutes to get the message that your body has had enough. If you eat too quickly, your stomach fills up before your brain knows you are full.

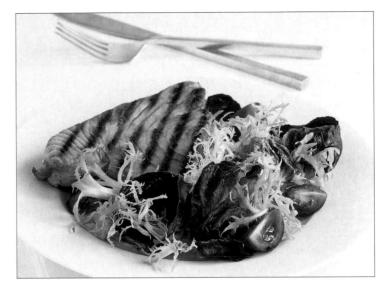

• Fill your plate with low-calorie, low-fat foods such as vegetables and salad.

• Throw away or freeze leftovers as soon as you've finished eating.

Above and below: A wide and varied selection of different foods, including fruit, vegetables and cereals, is always a good choice, and will keep hunger at bay.

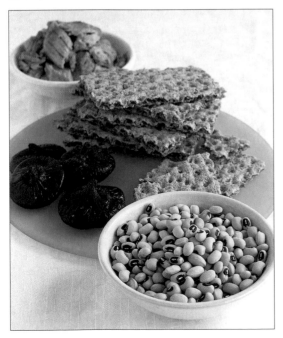

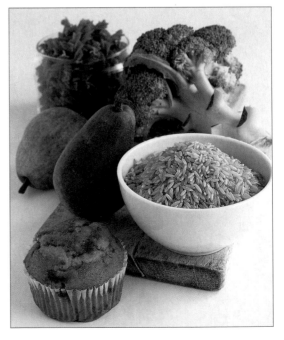

SLIMLINE SHOPPING

Bad planning can be the downfall of many diets, so make sure your fridge and store cupboards are stocked with a variety of healthy ingredients so that you'll always have the makings of a good nutritious meal or snack. Foods can be divided into five main groups – you need to eat some food from each group each day – but the key to a healthy diet is getting the balance right.

FRUIT AND VEGETABLES
These are the dieter's best friend: apart from being excellent providers of vitamins and minerals, they are also wonderfully low in both fat and calories. It's no coincidence that in Mediterranean countries, where people eat almost twice as much fruit and vegetables as we do, they live longer and healthier lives.

Don't just stick to the same old favourites – be adventurous and try something new. Look for recipes and ideas for new ways of cooking them – try poaching, baking or grilling fruits as an alternative to eating them raw.

Although fresh are best, frozen and canned fruits and vegetables and dried fruits are also useful. The vitamin C in both fruit and vegetables is easily destroyed during storage, preparation and cooking. To help preserve the vitamins, buy little and often. Buy from a shop that you know has a quick turnover and stores vegetables in a cool dark place, ideally for no more than three days. Boiling vegetables in large quantities of water can destroy up to 70 per cent of their vitamin C, so choose cooking methods that require little or no water. Aim to eat at least five servings a day.

STARCHY CARBOHYDRATES
This group, which includes bread, grains, rice, breakfast cereals, pasta and potatoes, should provide at least 50 per cent of our daily energy requirements. Unfortunately many people still believe that these foods are fattening, which is simply not the case. It's only when they are eaten with lots of fat – a rich sauce with pasta or thickly spread butter on bread – that they become so. Choose fibre-rich varieties, such as wholemeal bread and wholegrain cereals, whenever possible, as they provide slow-release energy, which helps keep blood sugar levels stable. High-fibre foods are more filling than their fibre-depleted counterparts: they will help you feel full more quickly and will stop you feeling hungry for longer.

Bread, rice, pasta, potatoes, couscous, polenta and bulgur wheat are all naturally low in fat. These are the foods to fill up on – at least half of the calories on your plate should come from starchy carbohydrate foods such as these. Be careful not to add too much fat when you cook them – 100g/3¾oz boiled potatoes contains just 80 calories but the same weight of chips contains 240 calories, which is three times as many.

PROTEIN FOODS
Meat, poultry, fish, eggs, nuts and pulses (peas, beans and lentils) are all excellent protein foods. Healthy eating recommendations suggest we should eat two to four servings from this group a day. To avoid unwanted calories always choose lean meat and poultry; white fish and pulses are also particularly good choices for people who are trying to lose weight.

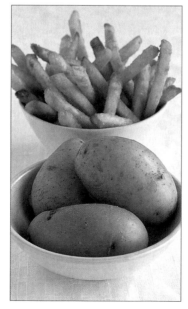

Above: Vegetables needn't be restricted to the tried and true – exotic varieties such as okra and sweet potato are increasingly available in local supermarkets.

Above: The above quantity of potatoes when boiled contains just 80 calories, while the same weight deep-fried has three times as many calories.

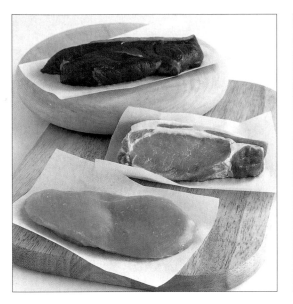

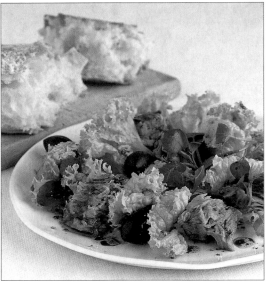

Above: Choose lean meat, such as venison, game, pork and chicken, whenever possible, all of which contain much less fat than red meats. Always trim away any visible fat before cooking, and choose a method of cooking that doesn't add any extra fat.

MEAT AND POULTRY

Red meat is an important source of iron, which can help prevent anaemia. Choose lean meat and trim away any visible fat before cooking. Pork, game and poultry all contain considerably less fat than lamb or beef.

FISH

Shellfish and white fish are both a particularly good choice for slimmers because they're extremely low in fat. Although oil-rich fish, such as salmon, mackerel and tuna, contain more fat, the type of fat they contain is particularly healthy and nutritionists suggest that we eat at least two servings of oil-rich fish a week. Canned fish is a useful ingredient to keep in the store cupboard for sandwiches or salads – choose fish canned in brine or water rather than oil.

EGGS

A good source of protein, eggs also provide vitamins A, B_1, B_2, B_{12} and folic acid. Egg yolks are a rich source of fat and cholesterol; however it is the amount and type of fat in the diet rather than the level of cholesterol in individual foods that will affect blood-cholesterol levels.

Because of the risk of salmonella poisoning, it is recommended that dishes containing raw or lightly cooked eggs should be avoided, particularly by young children, the elderly, pregnant women and anyone with an immune-deficiency disease.

NUTS

Chestnuts are the exception to the rule that nuts are high in fat. However, the type of fat that nuts contain is mainly the "healthier" unsaturated variety, and they also provide good amounts of vitamin E and protein. Therefore, providing they are used in small quantities, there is no reason why you should completely exclude nuts from your diet unless, of course, you have an allergy to them.

Above: Buy canned tuna, salmon and sardines that have been packed in brine, rather than oil. Lower in fat, canned fish is easily turned into a light and easily-prepared, Mediterranean-style salad.

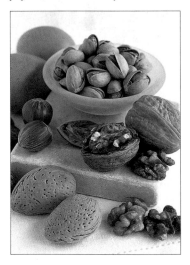

Above: Eggs and nuts, such as walnuts, almonds, hazelnuts and pistachios, are high in fat and should be eaten in moderation.

PULSES

An excellent source of low-fat protein, peas, beans and lentils are also high in fibre and provide useful amounts of vitamins and minerals. Pulses are economical, nutritious and incredibly versatile. You can use them to make dips such as hummus, soups, salads or curries, or to add to stews and casseroles. High-fibre foods are a good choice for slimmers because they help to satisfy the appetite and keep you feeling full for longer.

All dried beans (with the exception of lentils and split peas) should be soaked overnight in plenty of cold water. The next day, drain, rinse and place them in a saucepan with fresh water, bring to the boil and boil rapidly for 10 minutes (this will destroy the toxins that are naturally present in some types of bean), and then simmer until tender. Salt should not be added to the water until the end of the cooking time, as it will cause the skins to toughen.

MILK AND DAIRY PRODUCTS

Foods from this group are a major source of calcium, essential for strong bones. Many dairy products also contain large amounts of fat, most of which is saturated, and for this reason they should only be eaten in moderation. Choose reduced-fat varieties, such as skimmed and semi-skimmed milk, reduced-fat cheese and low-fat yogurts whenever possible.

Dairy products are a valuable source of calcium. They also provide useful amounts of protein and vitamins A, B_2, B_{12} and D. Choose reduced-fat dairy products whenever possible; they're just as nutritious as their full-fat cousins but contain fewer calories. Switching from full-fat to skimmed or semi-skimmed milk is a simple change – use skimmed milk to make sauces or custards and it is unlikely you will even notice the difference in taste.

Low-fat cheeses: There are an increasing number of low-fat cheeses available today. Interestingly, some traditional cheeses, such as Parmesan and Single Gloucester, were made with skimmed milk. The cream was skimmed off to use for cooking or to make butter. Most low-fat cheeses produced today, however, are the result of the increasing demand for low-fat products and the quality can vary, with an occasional lack in texture and depth of flavour. If you are not fond of low-fat cheeses, it can be more satisfying to choose a cheese with a strong flavour such as Parmesan or mature Cheddar for cooking, and just use less than you would if you were using a mild-flavoured cheese, thereby retaining taste but still reducing calories. Otherwise, try using a soft cheese for salads and sandwiches, as they have a high moisture content and therefore a lower percentage of fat than a harder cheese.

Other low-fat dairy products: Low-fat dairy products such as Quark, fromage frais and yogurt are a useful substitute for cream in sweet or savoury dishes.

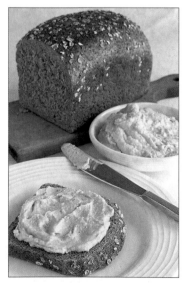

Above: For an excellent high-fibre snack, hummus is delicious spread on wholegrain bread or toast.

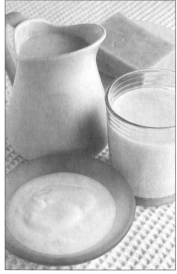

Above: From back, reduced-fat cheese, skimmed milk, semi-skimmed milk, and low-fat yogurt.

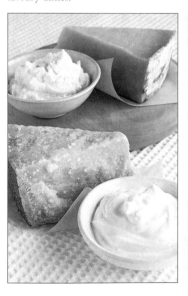

Above: From back, mature Cheddar, low-fat Quark, a large piece of fresh Parmesan and fromage frais.

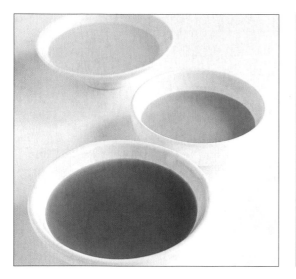

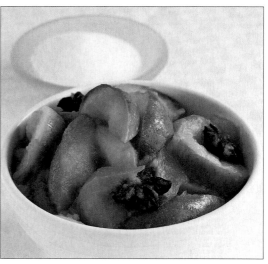

Above: From back, vegetable oil, walnut oil and extra virgin olive oil, believed by many to be best choice of all.

Above: If you really can't resist a touch of sweetness, use low-calorie sweeteners in desserts, such as stewed fruit.

FAT

Small amounts of fat are necessary in our diet to provide essential fatty acids and to allow the absorption of fat-soluble vitamins. However, a high-fat diet is known to increase the risk of heart disease, certain types of cancer and obesity. Current healthy eating recommendations suggest that fat should account for no more than 33 per cent of our total energy intake. For a woman on a 1,500-calorie a day diet, this amounts to 55g of fat per day.

Fat – the dieter's enemy: Weight for weight, fat provides twice as many calories as carbohydrate or protein and is the dieter's greatest concern. It is also thought that calories eaten as fat are more likely to be laid down as body fat than calories that come from protein or carbohydrate. But low-fat doesn't mean low taste. There are easy ways to trim the fat from your diet without giving up the foods you enjoy.

Whatever you spread on your bread – butter, margarine or low-fat spread – the message is to use it sparingly.

Low-fat spreads: Reduced- and low-fat spreads containing 40 per cent fat or more can be used for baking, for making sauces and for sautéing vegetables over a low heat. Spreads with less than 40 per cent fat are not suitable for cooking because of their high water content. Oils high in mono- or polyunsaturated fat such as olive oil, vegetable oil or nut oils are the best choice for salad dressings, sautéing vegetables and stir-frying.

SUGAR

It really does make sense to cut down on sugar where you can. Sugar simply provides "empty" calories – calories that provide nothing else in the way of protein, fibre, vitamins or minerals, and calories that most of us could do without. It's not necessary to avoid sugar completely; in fact, research carried out by Trinity College in Ireland found that people were more likely to abandon diets that demanded too strict a restriction of sugar and excluded all sweet foods.

You can accustom your taste buds to enjoy foods that are less sweet. It's not necessary to avoid all sugar on a weight-reducing diet, but 5ml/1 tsp

sugar contains 16 calories, which may not seem like very much, but it all mounts up. Brown sugar and honey have no nutritional advantage over white sugar although some people prefer the taste.

Low-calorie sweeteners: You can use low-calorie sweeteners as a substitute for sugar in hot drinks or for sweetening custard, stewed fruits and fruit fools. Sweeteners containing aspartame lose their sweetness at high temperatures, so it's best to add them at the end of cooking. Sweeteners based on saccharin or a mix of aspartame and asesulfame K are heat-stable and so can be used for cooking.

In baking, sugar adds bulk as well as sweetness. Low-calorie sweeteners don't provide the same bulk as sugar, so you shouldn't use low-calorie sweeteners for cakes, biscuits or meringues. Granular low-calorie sweeteners are about 10 times lighter than sugar – you can substitute the sweetener for sugar on a spoon for spoon basis but not weight for weight.

COOKING LIGHT

Just as important as the foods you choose is the way that you prepare them. Always use fresh, top-quality ingredients and choose cooking methods that use little or no fat. Use flavourings such as herbs, spices, lemon juice and mustard rather than fat to enhance the natural flavours of the food.

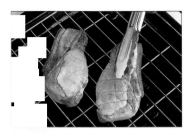

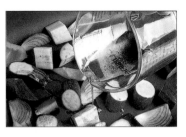

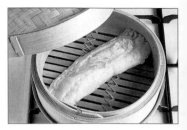

GRILLING
This requires little or no fat to be added during cooking and is much healthier than frying. It's a good method for tender cuts of meat, fish and succulent vegetables such as peppers and aubergine. Marinating food before grilling improves the flavour, and helps tenderize meat.

CHARGRILLING
A ridged iron griddle or pan allows the fat to drain away from the food. Lightly brush the food with oil to prevent it sticking to the pan and make sure the pan is really hot.

STIR-FRYING
This method gives food a good texture and flavour, and requires much less fat than either deep or shallow frying. It's a quick method of cooking and this helps preserve vitamins as well as the flavour. Make sure all the vegetables are cut into pieces of the same size so that they cook in the same amount of time.

ROASTING
Cook meat and poultry on a rack over a roasting tin to allow fat to drip underneath. Remove any fat before using the remaining juices to make gravy. Roasting is an excellent way of cooking vegetables such as aubergines, courgettes, onions, whole cloves of garlic and peppers. Cut the vegetables into large chunks and place in a large roasting tin, drizzle with a little olive oil and balsamic vinegar, season well and cook in the oven at 180°C/350°F/Gas 4 until tender.

POACHING
This is an excellent fat-free method for cooking fish, shellfish or poultry.

CASSEROLING
If casseroles are made the day before they are needed, they can be cooled and then refrigerated. Any excess fat can be skimmed off the surface before reheating. The flavours will also intensify overnight.

STEAMING
Special steamers are available in which water is boiled in the bottom compartment and the food is cooked in the compartment above. Alternatively, you can use a bamboo steamer or a metal basket-type steamer, which will fit into any size of saucepan. Steaming helps to retain flavour, colour and – most importantly – the water-soluble vitamins that are easily lost during other cooking methods, particularly boiling. Steaming is a good cooking method for fish.

EN PAPILLOTE
This refers to foods that are wrapped in greaseproof paper or foil and baked in the oven. It is a good method for cooking fruit, vegetables and delicate fish. No extra fat needs to be added when cooking by this method, but a couple of tablespoons of liquid, such as stock, wine or fruit juice should be added to create the steam that helps cook the food and keep it moist.

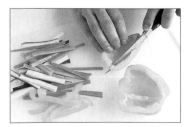

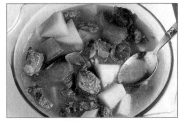

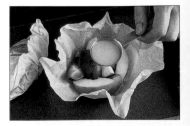

TRIMMING THE FAT

Fat provides twice as many calories as protein or carbohydrates. The most effective way of cutting the calories in your diet is therefore simple. It is to use low-fat ingredients, such as white fish and chicken, and low-fat alternatives wherever possible, such as reduced-fat cheese and skimmed milk.

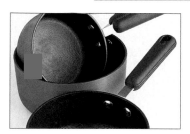

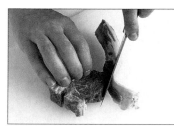

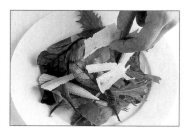

- Invest in a good, heavy-based non-stick pan and remember that oil expands once it gets hot, so when you're softening onions or vegetables you don't actually need as much oil as you might think. Use a vegetable or olive oil non-stick cooking spray for dishes that require light frying.
- Start with low-fat ingredients – white fish, shellfish, chicken and lean meat are all good choices.
- Choose low-fat cooking techniques such as poaching, braising, steaming, roasting, grilling or stir-frying.
- Marinades are a good way of adding extra flavour without fat.
- Don't be afraid to use strongly flavoured high-fat foods such as cheese and bacon; you only need to use small quantities to add a lot of flavour.
- To add flavour to dishes, use plenty of fresh herbs and spices in your cooking. Adding a squeeze of fresh lemon juice just before serving can also give your food a real lift.

- Always choose lean meat and trim away any visible fat before cooking. Remove the skin from poultry before eating.
- Bulk out savoury dishes by adding plenty of vegetables; they're low in calories and high in vitamins.
- Use reduced-fat alternatives such as reduced-fat cheese, skimmed milk, and low-fat yogurts where available.
- To make a reduced-fat white sauce, blend 15ml/1 tbsp cornflour with 30ml/2 tbsp cold water, and whisk this mixture into 300ml/½ pint/ 1¼ cups skimmed milk. Bring this to the boil and cook, stirring continuously, for 1 minute.
- Beware of high-fat salad dressings – 15ml/1 tbsp French dressing contains 97 calories and almost 11g fat, so use them in moderation.
- To make gravies and sauces creamy, add a little low-fat or Greek yogurt or fromage frais rather than cream. Stir in at the end of cooking to prevent curdling.

- Use cheese with a particularly strong flavour, such as a mature Cheddar, Parmesan or Stilton for making sauces or for garnishing and you will be able to use less. Adding a little mustard will also enhance the flavour.
- To reduce the fat in baked goods, such as muffins and cakes, replace half the fat with an equal quantity of something fruity, such as prune purée (see box below) or apple sauce.
- Go for fruit-based desserts and serve with a fruit coulis or puréed fruit, rather than cream or custard.

PRUNE PURÉE

Chop 115g/4oz stoned prunes and place in a blender along with 75ml/5 tbsp water. Process until smooth. Keep in an airtight container in the fridge for up to 3 days. Use for baking or stir into plain yogurt for a delicious dessert.

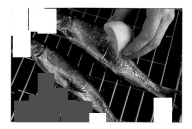

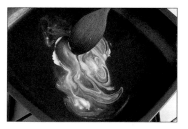

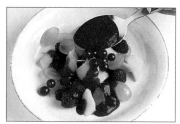

COUNTING THE CALORIES

Most of us eat fats in one form or another every day. In fact, its necessary to consume a small amount of fat to maintain a healthy and balanced diet, but almost everyone can afford to, and should, reduce their fat intake, particularly of saturated fats.

Dietary fats supply far more energy than all the other nutrients in our diet. By cutting down on fat, you can reduce your energy intake without affecting the other essential nutrients. The following charts will help you identify just which foods to avoid.

CALORIE AND FAT CONTENT IN DAIRY PRODUCTS PER 100G/3.5OZ

	Kcals/kJ	Fat(g)
double cream	449/1849	48
single cream	198/817	19
soured cream	205/861	20
whipping cream	373/1539	39
fromage frais (0% fat)	58/247	0.2
fromage frais (8% fat)	113/469	7.1
Greek yogurt (0% fat)	56/234	0
Greek yogurt, plain	115/477	9.1
low-fat natural yogurt	56/236	0.8
crème fraîche	380/1567	40
half-fat crème fraîche	195/815	15
Quark	74/309	0

CALORIE AND FAT CONTENT OF MILK PER 568ML/1 PINT

	Kcal/kJ	Fat(g)
full-fat	386/1615	22.8
semi-skimmed	269/1125	9.4
skimmed	193/807	0.6

CALORIE AND FAT CONTENT IN FATS, AND REDUCED-FAT SPREAD PER 100G/3.5OZ

	Kcals/kJ	Fat(g)
butter	737/3031	81
low-fat spread		
(40% fat)	388/1623	40
margarine	739/3039	81
reduced-fat spread		
(60% fat)	533/2230	60
very low-fat spread		
(20% fat)	183/765	20
cooking fat	891/3730	99

CALORIE AND FAT CONTENT OF CHEESES PER 100G/3.5OZ

	Kcals/kJ	Fat(g)
Parmesan	452/1880	33
Cheddar	412/1708	34
reduced-fat Cheddar	261/1091	15
Stilton	411/1719	35
Edam	333/1382	25
Gruyère	409/1711	33
Brie	319/1323	27
feta	250/1037	21
mozzarella	289/1209	21
ricotta	144/602	11
cottage cheese	98/410	4
cream cheese	439/1837	47.4

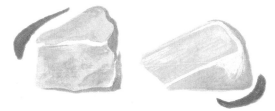

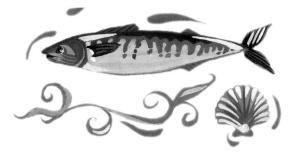

CALORIE AND FAT CONTENT IN MEAT AND MEAT PRODUCTS PER 100G/3.5OZ

	Kcals/kJ	Fat(g)
rump steak, lean and fat	174/726	10.1
rump steak, lean only	125/526	4.1
beef mince, raw	225/934	16.2
beef mince, raw, extra lean	174/728	9.6
bacon rasher, streaky, raw	276/1142	23.6
ham, premium	132/553	5.0
lamb, average, lean, raw	156/651	8.3
lamb chops, loin, lean and fat	277/1150	23.0
liver, lamb, raw	137/575	6.2
pork, average, lean, raw	123/519	4.0
pork chops, loin, lean and fat	270/1119	21.7
pork pie	376/1564	27.0
salami	491/2031	45.2
chicken fillet, raw	106/449	1.1
chicken roasted, meat and skin	218/910	12.5
turkey, meat only, raw	105/443	1.6
duck, meat only, raw	137/575	6.5
duck, roasted, meat, fat and skin	423/1750	38.1

CALORIE AND FAT CONTENT IN FISH AND SHELLFISH PER 100G/3.5OZ

	Kcals/kJ	Fat(g)
cod, battered and fried in oil	199/834	10.3
haddock, raw	81/345	0.6
kipper, baked	205/855	11.4
lemon sole, in crumbs and fried	216/904	13
trout, grilled	135/565	5.4
salmon, steamed	197/823	13
tuna, canned in brine	99/422	0.6
tuna, canned in oil	189/794	9.0
mackerel, smoked	354/1465	30.9
pilchards, canned in tomato sauce	126/531	5.4
squid, raw	66/278	1.5
crab, canned	77/326	0.5
mussels, boiled	87/366	2
prawns	99/418	0.9
shrimp, canned	94/398	1.2

LABEL LOW-DOWN

Reduced-calorie: contains 25 per cent fewer calories than the original calorie content. Beware, this does not necessarily mean the food in question is low in calories. For example, reduced-calorie mayonnaise contains 25 per cent fewer calories than standard mayonnaise but 25g/1oz still contains about 150 calories.
Low-calorie: contains fewer than 40 calories per serving or per 100g/3.5oz.
Reduced-fat: contains 22 per cent less fat than a similar full-fat product.
Low-fat: contains less than 5g fat per 100g/3.5oz.
Fat-free: virtually true. Fat-free products contain less than 0.1g fat per 100g/3.5oz.

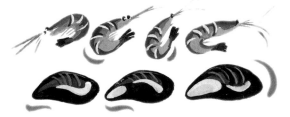

CEREALS, BAKING AND PRESERVES
PER 100G/3.5OZ

	Kcals/kJ	Fat(g)
bran flakes	31.8/135	1.9
wholewheat flakes	352/1498	2.7
sultana bran	303/1289	1.6
muesli	363/1540	5.9
bread roll, white	280/1192	2.3
wholemeal bread	215/914	2.5
wholemeal pitta bread	265/1127	1.2
croissant	360/1505	20.3
English muffin	310/1313	6.8
crumpet	199/846	1
shortbread	499/2087	26.1
digestive biscuit, plain	471/1978	20.9
doughnut, jam	336/1414	14.5
flapjack	484/2028	26.6
fruit cake, rich	341/1438	11
Madeira cake	393/1652	16.9
sponge cake, fatless	294/1245	6.1
chocolate, milk	529/2213	30.3
fruit jam	261/1116	0
honey	288/1205	0
lemon curd	283/1184	5.1
marmalade	261/1092	0
sugar, white	105/394	0

OILS AND DRESSINGS
PER 100G/3.5OZ

	Kcals/kJ	Fat(g)
olive oil	899/3761	99.9
coconut oil	899/3761	99.9
corn oil	899/3761	99.9
safflower oil	899/3761	99.9
French dressing	646/2702	72
mayonnaise	690/2816	76
reduced-fat mayonnaise	226/953	28.3

EGGS, RICE AND PASTA
PER 100G/3.5OZ

	Kcals/kJ	Fat(g)
egg	147/615	10.8
egg yolk	338/1414	30.5
egg white	100/418	0
white rice, uncooked	383/1630	3.6
brown rice, uncooked	356/1489	2.8
brown rice, boiled	141/589	1.1
pasta, plain	342/1456	1.6
pasta, wholemeal	324/1379	1.6
pasta, boiled	86/359	0.5
egg noodles, uncooked	392/1640	8.0

PULSES PER 100G/3.5OZ

	Kcals/kJ	Fat(g)
black-eyed beans, cooked	116/494	0.7
butter beans, canned	77/327	0.5
red kidney beans, canned	100/424	0.6
red lentils, cooked	100/424	0.4
chick-peas, canned	115/487	2.9
hummus	187/781	12.6

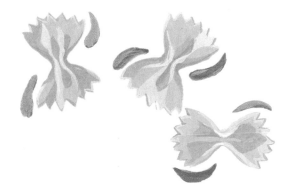

NUTS PER 100G/3.5OZ

	Kcals/kJ	Fat(g)
almonds	612/2560	55.8
walnuts	688/2888	68.5
Brazil nuts	682/2863	68.2
hazelnuts	650/2735	63.5
pistachio nuts	600/2510	56
chestnuts	172/719	2.8
pine nuts	688/2888	68.6
peanuts	608/2543	54
peanut butter, smooth	623/2606	53.7

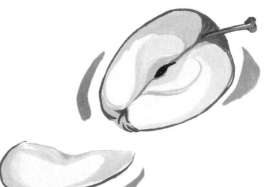

VEGETABLES PER 100G/3.5OZ

	Kcals/kJ	Fat(g)
spinach	25/103	0.8
broccoli	33/138	0.9
cabbage	26/109	0.4
cauliflower	34/142	0.9
aubergines	25/103	0.6
courgettes	18/75	0.4
tomatoes	16/66	0.3
lettuce	13/54	0
cucumber slice	16/66	0
fennel	12/50	0.2
leeks	22/93	0.5
peas	68/284	0.8
mangetouts, raw	32/136	0.2
mushrooms	13/55	0.5
onions	36/151	0.2
parsnips	64/271	1.1
carrots	23/96	0.4
potatoes:		
boiled new	75/314	0.3
baked	136/569	0.3
chips	189/793	6.7
roast	150/627	4.6
sweet potatoes	87/372	0.8

FRUIT PER 100G/3.5OZ

	Kcals/kJ	Fat(g)
apples	47/199	0.1
pears	40/169	0.1
avocados	190/795	19.5
bananas	95/403	0.3
grapefruit	30/125	0.1
oranges	37/158	0.1
apricots	30/125	0
peaches	33/138	0.1
strawberries	28/117	0
raspberries	24/100	0.4
dried mixed fruit	227/950	0.4
ready-to-eat dried apricots	160/670	0.6
ready-to-eat prunes	140/580	0.4

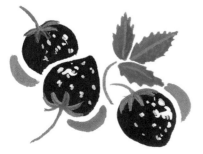

PUTTING IT ALL INTO PRACTICE

To achieve a steady, healthy weight loss you need to reduce your normal calorie intake by around 600 calories a day. For most women, between 1,200 and 1,500 calories a day should be sufficient, and for most men between 1,500 and 1,750 will probably be enough. In addition, it's important to spread your calorie allowance throughout the day – eating little and often will help both to maintain blood sugar levels and to resist the temptation to fall by the wayside and to snack or binge.

On a 1,200-calorie diet, allow 300 calories for breakfast, 350 for lunch, 400 for dinner, and 150 calories to used for snacks during the day. On a 1,500-calorie plan allow 300 for breakfast, 400 for lunch and 500 for dinner, plus 300 for snacks. If you prefer to count fat units, a 1,500-calorie diet allows 55g fat per day and 44g fat per day on a 1,200-calorie diet. All the recipes in this book are accompanied by a full nutritional analysis to help you create your own personal diet plan.

BREAKFAST

Many nutritionists are firmly convinced that breakfast is the most important meal of the day, and this is particularly true for anyone who is intent on watching their weight. Skipping breakfast in an attempt to save calories simply means that you're more likely to get hungry and start nibbling around mid-morning. Start the day with a low-fat, fibre-rich energy-boosting breakfast such as Luxury Muesli or Granola.

LUNCH

However busy you are, make sure that you find time to sit down and enjoy your lunch. Try to include at least two servings of fresh fruit and/or vegetables at lunchtime. Home-made soups, such as Garlic Soup, are both filling and nutritious, and are a good choice in the cold winter months.

EVENING MEAL

For most of us, this is usually the main meal of the day. It is time to unwind and relax, so make sure that you have a meal that you will really enjoy. Try stir-fried Chicken with Cashew Nuts

or Roasted Vegetables with Salsa Verde.

SNACKS

Whether you like to eat little and often or prefer to stick to three meals a day is a matter of personal preference, but many people find it helpful to have some snacks to hand in order to prevent energy dips mid-morning and mid-afternoon. The best in-between meal snack is a piece of fresh fruit. Alternatively, ready-to-eat dried fruits, such as apricots or prunes, are another

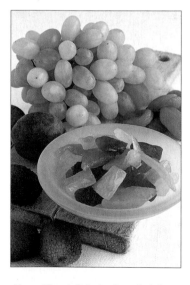

Above: There is little that beats fresh fruit for taste and ease in terms of healthy, low-fat snack food.

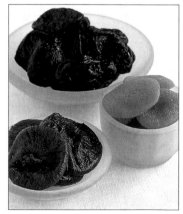

Above: Keep a selection of dried fruits as convenient store-cupboard ingredients to eat at any time.

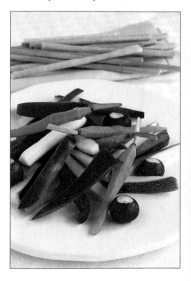

Above: Vegetable crudités make an ideal starter for a meal or as a snack. Serve with breadsticks or a low-fat dip.

DINING OUT ON A DIET

Just because you're on a diet
doesn't mean that you have to
forgo the pleasure of eating out.
Fortunately, most restaurants
nowadays offer a healthy choice as
part of their standard menu, even
if it is not highlighted as such on
the menu.

• If you want something special,
  ask. Don't be afraid to tell the
  waiter or waitress that you
  would like your vegetables
  served without butter or your
  fish without sauce, but make
  sure you do it when they take
  the order.
• Avoid calorie-laden starters such
  as avocado, pâté or anything
  deep fried. Choose melon and
  smoked salmon (above right),
  light soups, salad, or shellfish.
• Avoid creamy sauces, pastry and
  anything fried.
• Vegetarian options are not
  necessarily lower in calories –
  watch out especially for dishes
  that contain cheese or nuts.
• You don't have to miss out on
  dessert – just choose wisely.
  Fruit-based puddings, sorbets or
  meringue-based puddings, for
  example, are all good choices
  and won't pile on the calories.
• Be careful about how much you
  drink. It is well known that
  willpower dissolves in alcohol! A
  glass of wine may only contain
  about 100 calories but one glass
  can easily lead to another, and
  after a couple it's all too easy to
  forget all about your good
  intentions, which can have
  catastrophic results.
• Remember, one high calorie
  meal out won't ruin your diet. If
  you know you've eaten more
  than you should, be extra careful
  the following day.

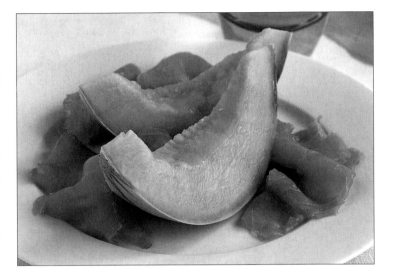

SNACKS AND TREATS

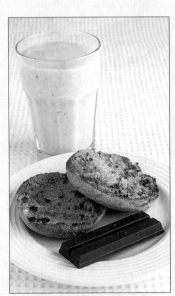

*Above: Hot muffins, milk drinks or
chocolate bars can be an acceptable treat
but preferably not altogether!*

50 calories
1 apple, orange or pear
10 strawberries
150ml/¼ pint/⅔ cup fruit juice
15ml/1 tbsp reduced-fat mayonnaise
1 chocolate-coated rice cake

100 calories
1 slice of malt loaf
4 fresh dates
6 ready-to-eat dried apricots
1 cappuccino or latte
1 banana
150ml/5fl oz glass of wine
1 pot virtually fat-free fruit yogurt
1 crumpet
1 oatcake topped with cottage cheese

150 calories
Honey and sesame seed bar
2 fingers of chocolate wafer biscuit
2 plain reduced-fat digestive biscuits
1 English fruit muffin
Banana smoothie: Place 1 small
banana, 75ml/5 tbsp natural low-fat
yogurt and 105ml/7 tbsp milk into a
blender and process until smooth.

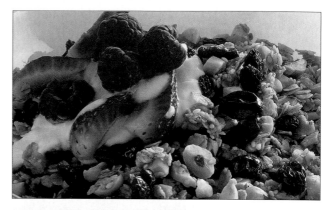

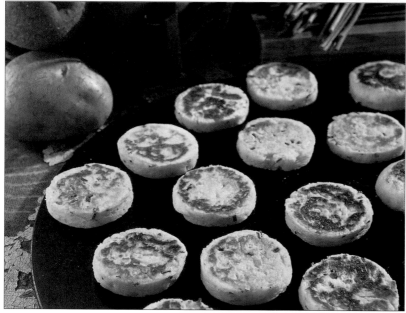

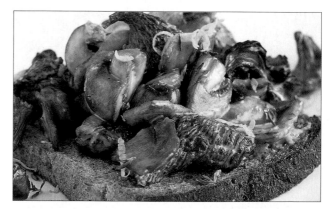

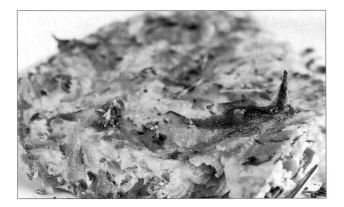

BREAKFAST

It is well known that breakfast is the most important meal of the day,

setting you up and charging your energy levels in preparation for all

the tasks that lie ahead of you. Choose from this tempting selection of

delicious options – such as fresh fruity smoothies, high-fibre

nutritious cereals, scones and muffins – and breakfast will not only be

a healthy part of your day, it will also be something that you look

forward to eagerly the moment you wake up.

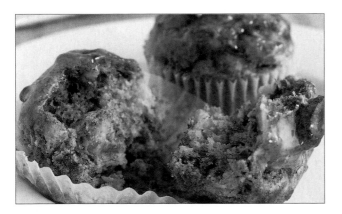

Totally Tropical

A delicious blend of
fruit and yogurt.

INGREDIENTS

Serves 2

1 ripe mango
250ml/8fl oz/1 cup
  pineapple juice
120ml/4fl oz/½ cup low-fat
  coconut yogurt
flaked coconut, to decorate

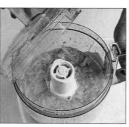

1 Peel and roughly chop
the mango. Place it and
the pineapple juice in a food
processor or blender. Process
until smooth.

2 Add the yogurt and
process for a further
30 seconds. Serve chilled,
decorated with a little flaked
coconut on top.

— NUTRITION NOTES —	
Per portion:	
Energy	143Kcals/598kJ
Fat, total	0.7g
saturated fat	0.3g
Protein	3.2g
Carbohydrate	33.3g
sugar, total	33.1g
Fibre – NSP	1.8g
Sodium	49mg

Cool Cranberry

For a quick fix of
vitamins, try this
refreshing smoothie.

INGREDIENTS

Serves 2

225g/8oz/2 cups strawberries
250ml/8fl oz/1 cup
  cranberry juice
120ml/4fl oz/½ cup low-fat
  strawberry yogurt

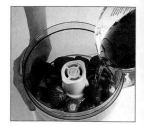

1 Place the strawberries
and cranberry juice in a
blender or food processor
and process for 1 minute or
until smooth.

2 Add the strawberry
yogurt and process for a
further 30 seconds. Serve
well chilled.

— NUTRITION NOTES —	
Per portion:	
Energy	121Kcals/506kJ
Fat, total	0.5g
saturated fat	0.2g
Protein	3.6g
Carbohydrate	27.5g
sugar, total	27.4g
Fibre – NSP	1.2g
Sodium	47mg

Banana Smoothie

A classic smoothie, this
one always delights.

INGREDIENTS

Serves 2

1 ripe pear and 1 banana
250ml/8fl oz/1 cup
  unsweetened apple juice
120ml/4fl oz/½ cup yogurt

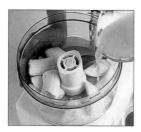

1 Peel and roughly chop
the pear and banana.
Place all the ingredients in a
blender or food processor,
and process until smooth.

— NUTRITION NOTES —	
Per portion:	
Energy	177Kcals/715kJ
Fat, total	0.9g
saturated fat	0.3g
Protein	3.2g
Carbohydrate	40.4g
sugar, total	39.5g
Fibre – NSP	1.5g
Sodium	44mg

— COOK'S TIP —
Add a pinch of ground cinnamon to this smoothie for extra flavour, if you wish.

Tropical Fruit Smoothie

Bright and breezy, this
will pick you up.

INGREDIENTS

Serves 2

3 kiwi fruits
200g/7oz fresh raspberries
250ml/8fl oz/1 cup passion
  fruit juice

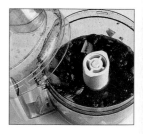

1 Peel and chop the kiwi
fruits then place all the
ingredients in a blender or
food processor, and process
until smooth.

— NUTRITION NOTES —	
Per portion:	
Energy	129Kcals/539kJ
Fat, total	0.1g
saturated fat	0.1g
Protein	3.4g
Carbohydrate	27.3g
sugar, total	27.0g
Fibre – NSP	4.1g
Sodium	29mg

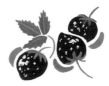

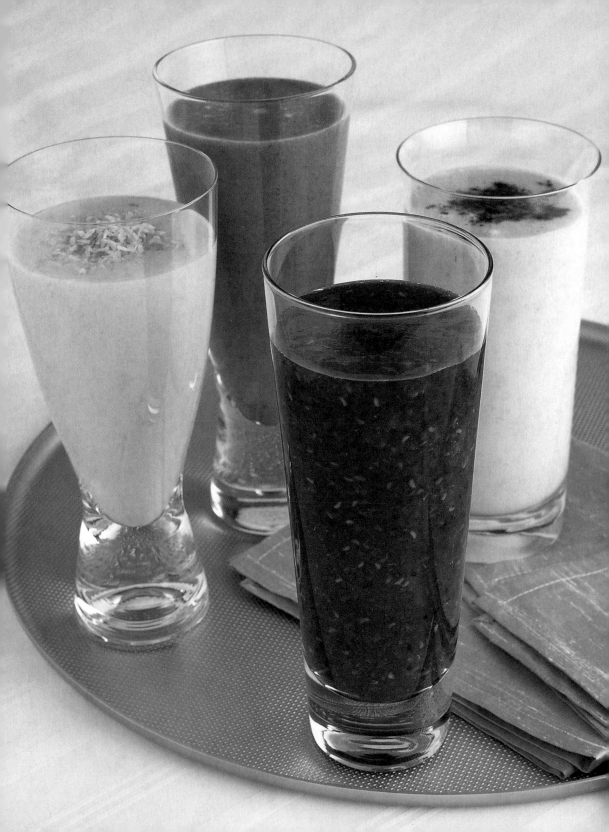

Luxury Muesli

Eating a bowl of muesli for breakfast provides you with a low-fat, high-fibre start. It will forestall those mid-morning munchies, which can prove the downfall of someone trying to lose weight.

INGREDIENTS

Serves 12
50g/2oz/½ cup sunflower seeds
25g/1oz/¼ cup pumpkin seeds
115g/4oz/1 cup porridge oats
115g/4oz/heaped 1 cup wheat flakes
115g/4oz/heaped 1 cup barley flakes
115g/4oz/1 cup raisins
115g/4oz/1 cup chopped hazelnuts,
 lightly roasted
115g/4oz/½ cup unsulphured dried
 apricots, chopped
50g/2oz/2 cups dried apple
 slices, halved
25g/1oz/⅓ cup desiccated coconut

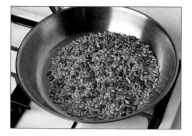
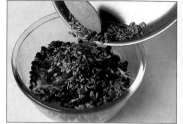

1 Put the sunflower and pumpkin seeds in a dry frying pan and cook over a medium heat for 3 minutes until golden, tossing the seeds regularly to prevent them burning. Allow to cool. Place the remaining ingredients in a large, clean bowl.

2 Add the seeds, mix together well and store in an airtight container.

---- COOK'S TIP ----

Serve the muesli in a long glass layered with fresh raspberries and fromage frais. Soak the muesli first in a little water or fruit juice in order to soften it slightly.

——— NUTRITION NOTES ———	
Per portion:	
Energy	262Kcals/1097kJ
Fat, total	11.3g
saturated fat	2.1g
Protein	3.6g
Carbohydrate	35.4g
sugar, total	17.2g
Fibre – NSP	5.9g
Sodium	186mg

Granola

Serve with semi-skimmed milk or natural live yogurt and fresh fruit for an excellent and nutritious start to the day.

INGREDIENTS

Serves 6
115g/4oz/1 cup porridge oats
115g/4oz/1 cup jumbo oats
50g/2oz/⅓ cup sunflower seeds
25g/1oz/2 tbsp sesame seeds
50g/2oz/½ cup hazelnuts, roasted
25g/1oz/¼ cup almonds,
 roughly chopped
50ml/2fl oz/¼ cup sunflower oil
50ml/2fl oz/¼ cup clear honey
50g/2oz/⅓ cup raisins
50g/2oz/⅓ cup dried sweetened
 cranberries

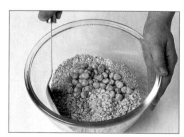

1 Preheat the oven to 140°C/275°F/ Gas 1. Mix together the oats, seeds and nuts in a bowl.

2 Heat the oil and honey in a large saucepan until melted, then remove the pan from the heat. Add the oat mixture and stir well. Spread out on one or two baking sheets.

3 Bake the oats and honey mixture for about 50 minutes until crisp, stirring occasionally to prevent the mixture sticking. Remove from the oven and mix in the raisins and cranberries. Leave to cool, then store the granola in an airtight container.

——— NUTRITION NOTES ———	
Per portion:	
Energy	280Kcals/1174kJ
Fat, total	19.8g
saturated fat	2g
Protein	5.2g
Carbohydrate	21.6g
sugar, total	16.8g
Fibre – NSP	2.3g
Sodium	195mg

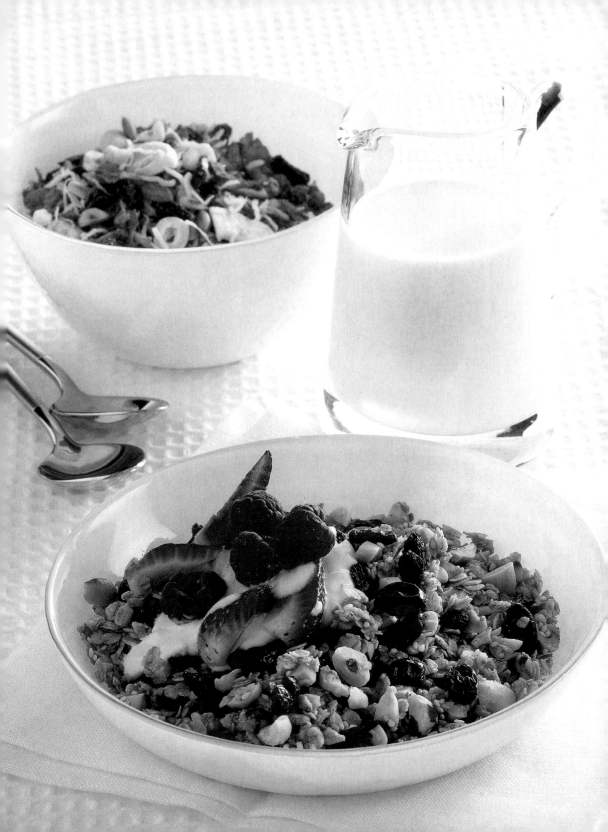

Chive and Potato Scones

These little chive and potato scones should be fairly thin, soft on the inside and crisp and golden brown on the outside. They are a treat as a delicious and healthy breakfast. The quantities given here make enough to serve to overnight guests as a special Sunday brunch.

Ingredients

Makes 20
450g/1lb potatoes
115g/4oz/1 cup plain flour, sifted
30ml/2 tbsp olive oil
30ml/2 tbsp snipped chives
salt and freshly ground black pepper
low-fat spread, for topping
   (optional)

1 Cook the potatoes in a saucepan of boiling salted water for 20 minutes, then drain. Return the potatoes to a clean pan and mash them. Preheat a griddle or heavy-based frying pan.

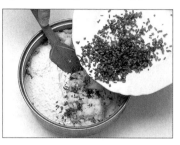

2 Add the flour, the olive oil and the chives to the hot mashed potato in the pan, and season with a little salt and pepper. Mix to a soft dough.

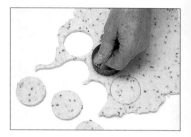

3 Roll out the prepared dough on a well-floured surface to a thickness of about 5mm/¼in and stamp out rounds with a 5cm/2in plain pastry cutter. Lightly grease the griddle or heavy-based frying pan.

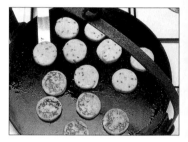

4 Cook the scones, in batches, on the hot griddle or frying pan for about 10 minutes. Using a metal spatula, turn each scone once, cooking until they are golden brown on both sides. Keep the heat low and do not allow them to burn. Top the scones with a little low-fat spread, if you like, and serve them immediately, while still piping hot.

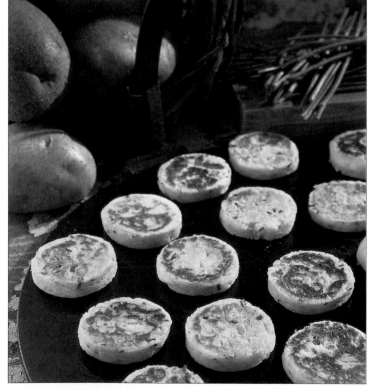

Nutrition Notes	
Per portion:	
Energy	25Kcals/104kJ
Fat, total	1.2g
saturated fat	0.2g
Protein	0.9g
Carbohydrate	8.1g
sugar, total	0.4g
Fibre – NSP	0.4g
Sodium	2.6mg

Banana and Walnut Muffins

Deliciously moist and fruity, these muffins provide a high-fibre, low-fat alternative to croissants or Danish pastries for a breakfast treat that won't leave you feeling guilty.

INGREDIENTS

Makes 6

115g/4oz/1 cup wholemeal flour
25g/1oz/¼ cup wheatgerm
45ml/3 tbsp caster sugar
10ml/2 tsp baking powder
75g/3oz/¾ cup chopped walnuts
1 large egg, beaten
50ml/2fl oz/¼ cup milk
50ml/2fl oz/¼ cup sunflower oil
2 ripe bananas, about 225g/8oz
   when peeled
apricot jam, to glaze

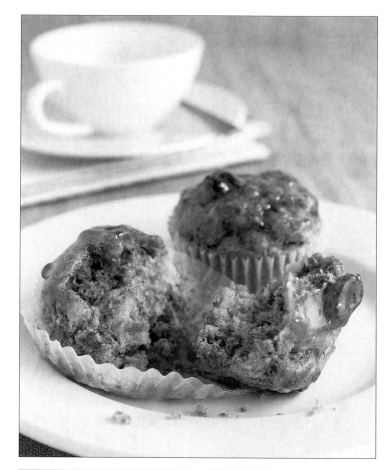

1 Line 6 muffin tins with individual paper muffin cases or grease the tins well. Preheat the oven to 200°C/400°F/Gas 6.

2 In a large mixing bowl, mix together the flour, wheatgerm, sugar, baking powder and walnuts. In a separate bowl, whisk together the egg, milk and sunflower oil. Then pour all the liquid ingredients into the flour mixture and stir until blended.

3 Roughly mash the ripe bananas, and stir these into the flour and egg mixture. Take particular care not to overmix.

--- NUTRITION NOTES ---

Per portion:

Energy	294Kcals/1230kJ
Fat, total	16.3g
saturated fat	1.9g
Protein	7.6g
Carbohydrate	31.7g
sugar, total	17.3g
Fibre – NSP	3.2g
Sodium	181mg

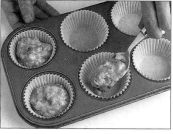

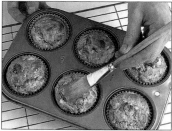

4 Fill each muffin case two-thirds full. Bake for 20–25 minutes, or until a skewer inserted into the centre comes out clean. Transfer the muffins to a wire rack to cool slightly.

5 Brush the tops of the muffins with a little warm apricot jam and serve immediately.

Mushrooms with Bacon, Thyme and Lemon

Served with slices of toast, these mushrooms are great for breakfast but you can also serve them with pasta or polenta for a light lunch.

INGREDIENTS

Serves 2

10g/¼oz dried mushrooms
15ml/1 tbsp olive oil
75g/3oz rindless lean smoked bacon, roughly chopped
175g/6oz brown cap mushrooms, roughly chopped
200ml/7fl oz/scant 1 cup chicken stock
5ml/1 tsp fresh thyme, chopped, plus extra to garnish
45ml/3 tbsp reduced fat crème fraîche
finely grated zest of 1 lemon
salt and freshly ground black pepper
slices of wholemeal toast, to serve

1 Place the dried mushrooms in a large bowl, pour over enough boiling water to cover, then leave to soak for about 15 minutes. Drain the soaked mushrooms, pat dry and, using a sharp knife, roughly chop them into equal, bite-size pieces.

NUTRITION NOTES	
Per portion:	
Energy	183Kcals/765kJ
Fat, total	15.4g
saturated fat	5.3g
Protein	9.7g
Carbohydrate	1.6g
sugar, total	0.3g
Fibre – NSP	1.6g
Sodium	647mg

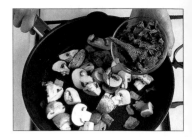

2 Heat the oil in a frying pan, add the bacon and cook, stirring occasionally, for 5 minutes or until beginning to brown. Add the fresh and dried mushrooms and continue to cook for a further 5 minutes.

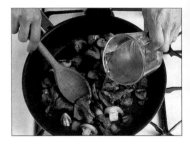

3 Add the chicken stock, thyme and seasoning, reduce the heat slightly and cook for 10–15 minutes or until the liquid has reduced and is thick and syrupy.

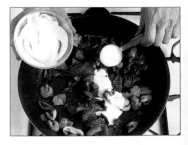

4 Stir in the crème fraîche and lemon zest. Scoop on to the slices of toast, garnish with a little more fresh thyme and serve immediately.

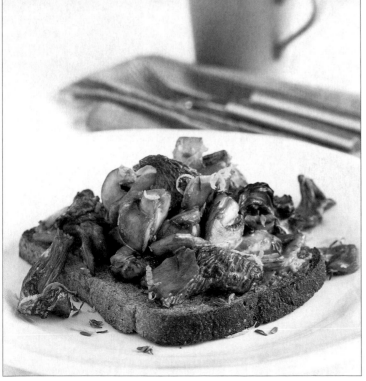

Carrot and Courgette Frittata

Frittata is the Italian version of an omelette. The filling ingredients are set in the eggs as they cook, rather than being served in the middle of a folded omelette. If you want something a little special, try a combination of smoked salmon and asparagus tips, for a wonderful, rich flavour.

INGREDIENTS

Serves 2
1 carrot
1 courgette
4 eggs, beaten
60ml/4 tbsp skimmed milk
15ml/1 tbsp olive oil
30ml/2 tbsp grated reduced-fat
   Cheddar cheese (optional)
salt and freshly ground black pepper

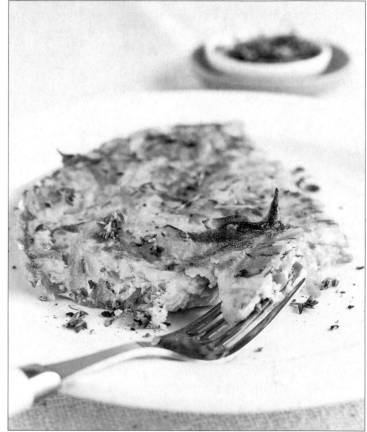

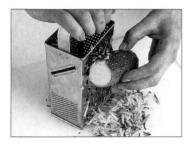

1 Grate the carrot and courgette. In a clean bowl, whisk together the eggs, milk and seasoning.

NUTRITION NOTES	
Per portion:	
Energy	251Kcals/1050kJ
Fat, total	19g
saturated fat	4.7g
Protein	16.8g
Carbohydrate	3.4g
sugar, total	3.2g
Fibre – NSP	1.2g
Sodium	191mg

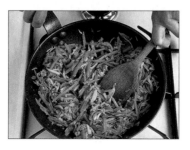

2 Preheat the grill. Heat the olive oil in a small non-stick frying pan. Add the grated carrot and courgette, and cook the vegetables over a medium heat, stirring occasionally, for 2–3 minutes.

3 Pour in the egg mixture, then sprinkle over the cheese, if using, and cook for 4 minutes or until the base is just set. Transfer to the grill and cook for a further 4 minutes or until just firm to the touch.

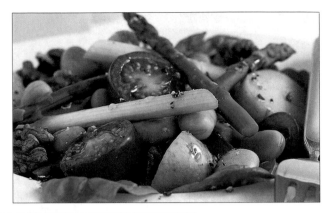

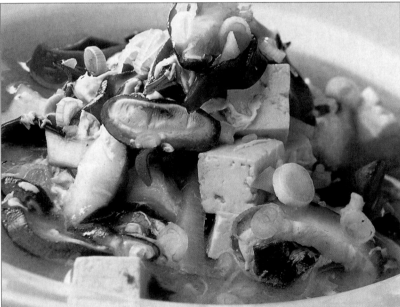

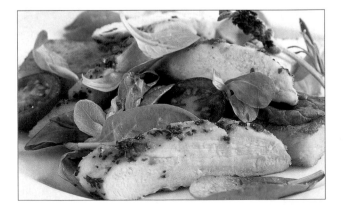

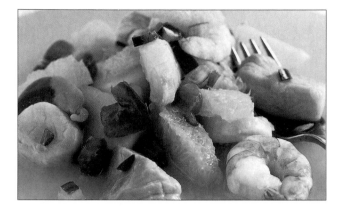

STARTERS AND
LIGHT MEALS

*Sometimes it's just not possible to prepare a full meal, but quick-and-
easy doesn't necessarily mean lacking in flavour or nutrition. This
chapter has many suggestions for delicious dishes such as soups,
crunchy vegetable omelettes, or salads, which you can serve either as a
starter or a light meal. Try Clam and Pasta Soup, for example,
Tuna Carpaccio, or Baked Sweet Potato Salad.*

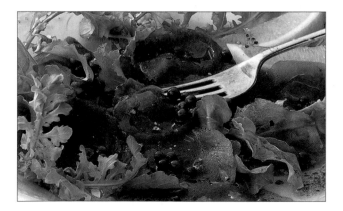

Clam and Pasta Soup

Subtly sweet and spicy, this soup is substantial enough to be served on its own for lunch or supper.

INGREDIENTS

Serves 4

30ml/2 tbsp olive oil
1 onion, finely chopped
leaves from 1 fresh thyme sprig,
   chopped, plus extra to garnish
2 garlic cloves, crushed
5–6 fresh basil leaves, torn, plus extra
   to garnish
1.5–2.5ml/¼–½ tsp crushed red chillies
1 litre/1¾ pints/4 cups fish stock
350ml/12fl oz/1½ cups passata
5ml/1 tsp granulated sugar
90g/3½oz/scant 1 cup frozen peas
65g/2½oz/⅔ cup small pasta shapes
225g/8oz frozen shelled clams, thawed,
   or bottled clams in their shells
salt and freshly ground black pepper

1 Heat the oil in a large saucepan, add the onion and cook gently for about 5 minutes until softened. Add the thyme, then stir in the garlic, basil leaves and red chillies to taste.

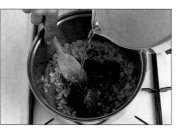

2 Add the stock, passata and sugar to the saucepan, with salt and pepper to taste. Bring to the boil, then lower the heat and simmer gently, stirring occasionally, for about 15 minutes. Add the frozen peas and cook for a further 5 minutes.

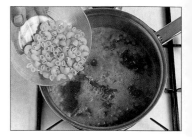

3 Add the pasta to the stock mixture and bring to the boil, stirring. Lower the heat and simmer, stirring frequently, until the pasta is only just *al dente* – about 5 minutes or according to the instructions on the packet.

4 Reduce the heat to low, add the frozen or bottled clams and heat through for 2–3 minutes. Taste for seasoning. Serve hot in warmed bowls, garnished with the extra fresh basil and thyme.

COOK'S TIP

Frozen shelled clams are available at good fishmongers and supermarkets, but if you can't get them, use bottled or canned clams in natural juice (not vinegar).

NUTRITION NOTES

Per portion:

Energy	209Kcals/874kJ
Fat, total	6.7g
saturated fat	0.9g
Protein	15.6g
Carbohydrate	22.9g
sugar, total	6.5g
Fibre – NSP	2.8g
Sodium	1253mg

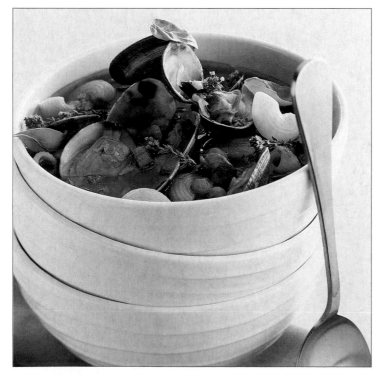

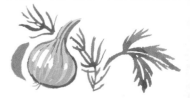

Garlic Soup

This is a simple and satisfying Mediterranean soup, and will keep the hunger pangs at bay. Paprika, cumin and saffron come together to create a wonderful aroma and taste.

INGREDIENTS

Serves 4

30ml/2 tbsp olive oil
4 large garlic cloves, peeled
4 slices French bread, 5mm/¼in thick
15ml/1 tbsp paprika
1 litre/1¾ pints/4 cups beef stock
1.5ml/¼ tsp ground cumin
pinch of saffron strands
4 eggs
salt and freshly ground black pepper
chopped fresh parsley,
    to garnish

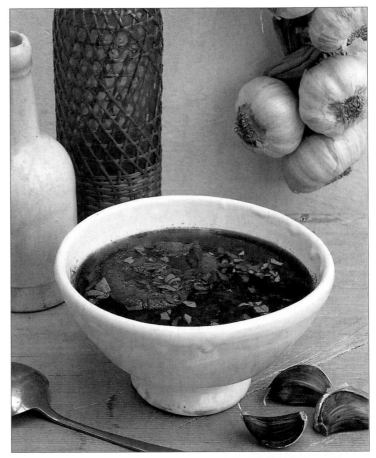

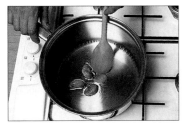

1 Preheat the oven to 230°C/450°F/ Gas 8. Heat the oil in a large pan. Add the whole garlic cloves and cook until golden. Remove and set aside. Fry the bread in the oil on both sides until golden, then set aside.

2 Add the paprika to the pan, and fry for a few seconds. Stir in the beef stock, cumin and saffron, then add the reserved garlic, crushing the cloves with the back of a wooden spoon. Season with salt and pepper, then cook for about 5 minutes.

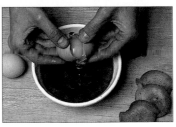

3 Ladle the soup into four ovenproof bowls and break an egg into each. Place the slices of fried bread on top of the egg and place in the oven for about 3–4 minutes, until the eggs are set. Sprinkle with parsley and serve at once.

NUTRITION NOTES	
Per portion:	
Energy	176Kcals/736kJ
Fat, total	12.1g
saturated fat	2.6g
Protein	10.4g
Carbohydrate	6.8g
sugar, total	0.3g
Fibre – NSP	0.3g
Sodium	677mg

COOK'S TIP

Saffron is the most expensive spice in the world, but very little of this subtle ingredient is needed to give both flavour and colour to a dish, as here.

Hot-and-sour Soup

This spicy, warming soup, low in fat but high in flavour, is a good choice for anyone watching their weight. Serve as a starter or as a light main course.

INGREDIENTS

Serves 4

10g/¼oz dried cloud ears
8 fresh shiitake mushrooms
75g/3oz tofu (bean curd)
50g/2oz/½ cup sliced, drained, canned bamboo shoots
900ml/1½ pints/3½–4 cups vegetable stock
15ml/1 tbsp caster sugar
45ml/3 tbsp rice vinegar
15ml/1 tbsp light soy sauce
1.5ml/¼ tsp chilli oil
2.5ml/½ tsp salt
large pinch of ground white pepper
15ml/1 tbsp cornflour
15ml/1 tbsp cold water
1 egg white
5ml/1 tsp sesame oil
2 spring onions, cut into fine rings

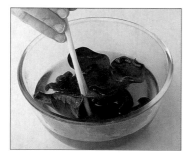

1 Soak the cloud ears in hot water for 30 minutes or until soft. Drain, trim off and discard the hard base from each and chop the cloud ears roughly.

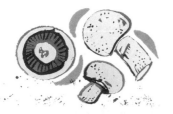

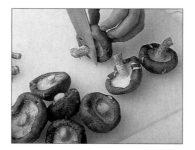

2 Remove and discard the stalks from the shiitake mushrooms. Cut the caps into thin strips. Cut the tofu into 1cm/½in cubes and shred the bamboo shoots finely.

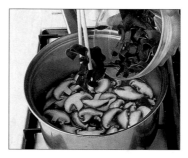

3 Place the stock, mushrooms, tofu, bamboo shoots and cloud ears in a pan. Bring the stock to the boil, lower the heat and simmer for 5 minutes.

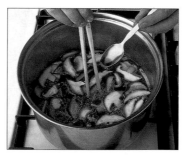

4 Stir in the sugar, vinegar, soy sauce, chilli oil, salt and pepper. Mix the cornflour to a paste with the water. Add the mixture to the soup, stirring constantly until it thickens slightly.

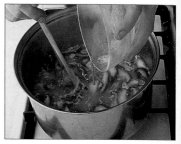

5 Lightly beat the egg white, then pour it slowly into the soup in a steady stream, stirring constantly. Cook, stirring, until the egg white changes colour.

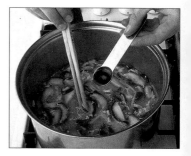

6 Add the sesame oil to the pan just before serving. Ladle the soup into heated bowls and decorate each portion with a few sliced spring onion rings. Serve piping hot.

NUTRITION NOTES	
Per portion:	
Energy	90Kcals/376kJ
Fat, total	2.2g
saturated fat	0.3g
Protein	5g
Carbohydrate	13.4g
sugar, total	5.3g
Fibre – NSP	0.4g
Sodium	807mg

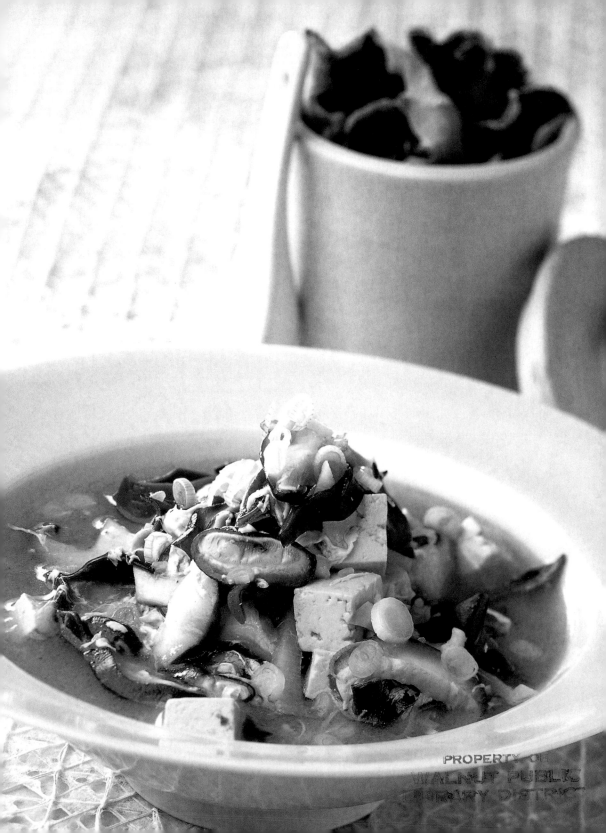

PROPERTY OF
WALNUT PUBLIC
LIBRARY DISTRICT

Cannellini Bean and Rosemary Toasts

Cannellini beans are high in protein and low in fat. This sophisticated version of beans on toast makes an ideal brunch or light lunch.

INGREDIENTS

Serves 6

150g/5oz/⅔ cup dried cannellini beans
5 tomatoes
45ml/3 tbsp olive oil, plus extra
   for drizzling
2 sun-dried tomatoes in oil, drained
   and finely chopped
1 garlic clove, crushed
30ml/2 tbsp chopped fresh rosemary
salt and freshly ground block pepper
handful of fresh basil leaves, to garnish

To serve

12 slices Italian-style bread, such
   as ciabatta
1 large garlic clove, halved

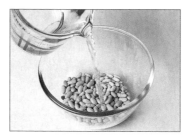

1 Soak the beans in a large bowl of water overnight. Drain and rinse the beans, then cover with fresh water in a saucepan. Bring to the boil and boil rapidly for 10 minutes. Reduce the heat and simmer for 50–60 minutes or until tender. Drain and set aside.

> ——— COOK'S TIP ———
>
> Canned beans may be used if you wish; use 275g/10oz/2 cups and add in step 3.

2 Meanwhile, place the tomatoes in a bowl, cover with boiling water, leave for 30 seconds, then peel, seed and chop the flesh. Heat the oil in a frying pan, add the fresh and sun-dried tomatoes, garlic and rosemary. Cook for 2 minutes until the tomatoes begin to break down and soften.

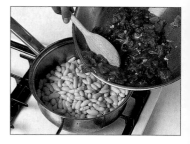

3 Add the tomato mixture to the cannellini beans, season and stir.

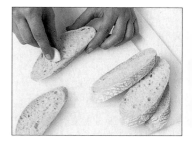

4 To serve, rub the cut sides of the bread with the garlic clove, then toast lightly. Spoon the cannellini bean mixture on top of the toast, sprinkle with basil and drizzle with olive oil.

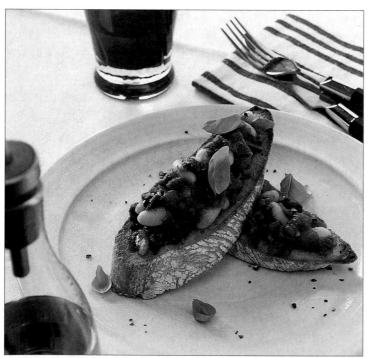

> ——— NUTRITION NOTES ———
>
> Per portion:
>
> | | |
> |---|---|
> | Energy | 320Kcals/1338kJ |
> | Fat, total | 9.1g |
> | saturated fat | 1.46g |
> | Protein | 12.4g |
> | Carbohydrate | 50.2g |
> | sugar, total | 4.16g |
> | Fibre – NSP | 5.6g |
> | Sodium | 415mg |

Coriander Omelette Parcels

Crunchy fresh vegetables flavoured with ginger, chillies and tangy coriander, and wrapped in a thin omelette make a tasty and healthy meal.

INGREDIENTS

Serves 4

30ml/2 tbsp groundnut oil
1cm/½in piece fresh root ginger, finely grated
1 large garlic clove, crushed
2 red chillies, seeded and finely sliced
4 spring onions, sliced diagonally
130g/4½oz broccoli, cut into small florets and blanched for 2 minutes
175g/6oz/3 cups shredded pak choi
50g/2oz/2 cups fresh coriander leaves, plus extra to garnish
115g/4oz/½ cup beansprouts
45ml/3 tbsp black bean sauce
4 eggs, lightly beaten
salt and freshly ground black pepper

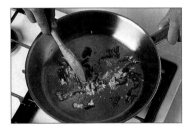

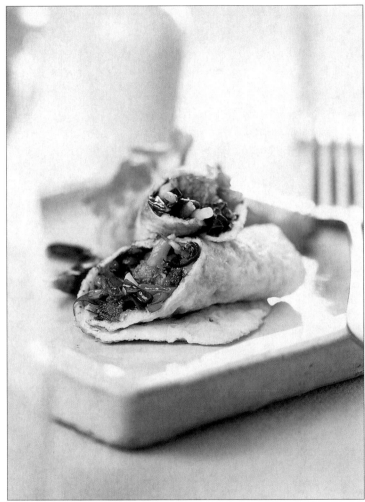

1 Heat 15ml/1 tbsp of the oil in a frying pan or wok. Add the ginger, garlic and half the chillies, and stir-fry for 1 minute. Add the spring onions, blanched broccoli and pak choi, and stir-fry for 2 minutes more, tossing all the vegetables continuously to prevent them sticking and to cook them evenly.

2 Chop three-quarters of the coriander and add to the pan. Add the beansprouts and stir-fry for about 1 minute, then add the black bean sauce and heat through for 1 minute more. Remove the pan from the heat and keep warm.

3 Season the eggs well. Heat a little of the remaining oil in a pan and add a quarter of the beaten egg. Swirl the egg until it covers the base of the pan, then scatter over a quarter of the reserved coriander leaves. Cook until set and turn out on to a plate. Make three more omelettes in the same way.

4 Spoon the vegetable stir-fry on to the omelettes and roll up. Serve garnished with coriander leaves.

NUTRITION NOTES	
Per portion:	
Energy	178Kcals/744kJ
Fat, total	12.6g
saturated fat	3g
Protein	11.3g
Carbohydrate	5.3g
sugar, total	4.5g
Fibre – NSP	2.7g
Sodium	370mg

Yellow Tomato and Orange Pepper Salsa

Serve this sunny salsa with plain grilled meats or fish. It will add plenty of flavour – and colour – to the finished dish without piling on the calories.

INGREDIENTS

Serves 4
4 yellow tomatoes
1 orange pepper
4 spring onions, plus extra to garnish
handful of fresh coriander leaves
juice of 1 lime
salt and freshly ground black pepper

1 Halve the tomatoes and scoop out the seeds, using a teaspoon, and discard. Finely chop the flesh.

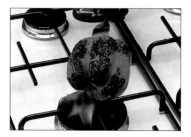

2 Spear the pepper on a metal fork and turn it in a gas flame for 1–2 minutes until the skin blisters, or place it under a hot grill and turn frequently.

3 Peel off and discard the skin. Remove the core and scrape out the seeds. Finely chop the flesh.

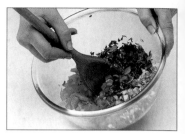

4 Finely chop the spring onions and coriander, then mix both with the pepper and tomato flesh.

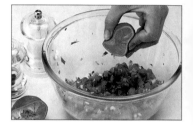

5 Squeeze over the lime juice and add salt and pepper to taste. Toss well to mix. Finally, transfer the prepared salsa to a serving bowl and chill until you are ready to serve. Garnish with a few fine shreds of spring onion.

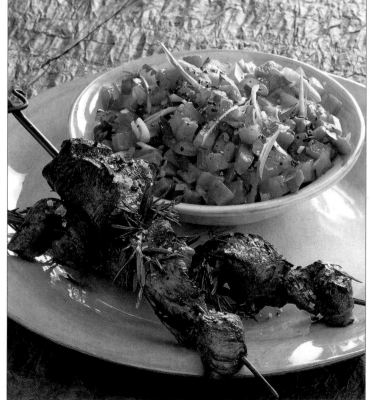

NUTRITION NOTES	
Per portion:	
Energy	26Kcals/108kJ
Fat, total	0.4g
saturated fat	0.1g
Protein	1.1g
Carbohydrate	4.8g
sugar, total	4.7g
Fibre – NSP	1.4g
Sodium	8.2mg

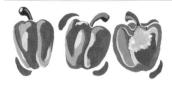

Ceviche

Raw fish is marinated in citrus juices, whose acidity "cooks" the fish without the need for any oil.

INGREDIENTS

Serves 6

350g/12oz/3 cups medium cooked prawns
350g/12oz/3 cups scallops, removed from their shells, with corals intact if possible
175g/6oz tomatoes, diced
1 mango, weighing about 175g/6oz, diced
1 red onion, finely chopped
350g/12oz salmon fillet
1 fresh red chilli
juice of 8 limes
30ml/2 tbsp sugar
2 pink grapefruits
3 oranges
4 limes
salt and freshly ground black pepper

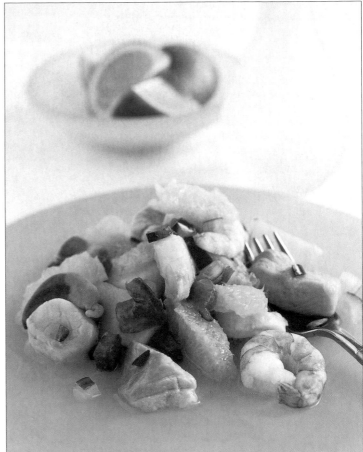

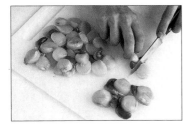

1 Peel the prawns and cut the scallops into 1cm/½in dice. In a bowl, mix together the diced tomatoes, mango and red onion.

NUTRITION NOTES	
Per portion:	
Energy	330Kcals/1380kJ
Fat, total	8.2g
saturated fat	1.5g
Protein	40.4g
Carbohydrate	25.3g
sugar, total	23g
Fibre – NSP	3.2g
Sodium	1067mg

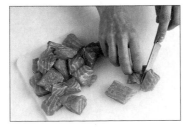

2 Cut the salmon into small pieces. Dice the chilli, and mix with the fish, tomato and mango. Add the lime juice, sugar and seasoning. Stir and leave to marinate for 3 hours.

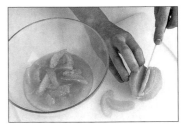

3 Segment the grapefruit, oranges and limes. Drain off as much excess lime juice as possible and mix the fruit segments into the marinated ingredients. Season to taste and serve.

Grilled Chicken Salad with Lavender

Lavender may seem like an odd salad ingredient, but its delightful scent has a natural affinity with sweet garlic, orange and wild herbs. Make the most of natural flavourings, which can add interest to a meal without the need to add fattening ingredients.

INGREDIENTS

Serves 6

4 boneless skinless chicken breasts
900ml/1½ pints/3¾ cups light
  chicken stock
175g/6oz/1 cup fine polenta
50g/2oz/4 tbsp butter
450g/1lb young spinach
175g/6oz lamb's lettuce
8 fresh lavender sprigs
8 small tomatoes, halved
salt and freshly ground black pepper

For the lavender marinade

6 stems fresh lavender
10ml/2 tsp finely grated orange zest
2 garlic cloves, crushed
10ml/2 tsp clear honey
30ml/2 tbsp olive oil
10ml/2 tsp chopped fresh thyme
10ml/2 tsp chopped fresh marjoram
salt

NUTRITION NOTES

Per portion:

Energy	332Kcals/1383kJ
Fat, total	11.3g
saturated fat	5.2g
Protein	30g
Carbohydrate	26.6g
sugar, total	4.13g
Fibre – NSP	2.8g
Sodium	603mg

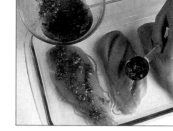

1 To make the marinade, strip the lavender flowers from the stems and combine with the orange zest, garlic, honey and salt. Add the olive oil and herbs. Slash the chicken breasts deeply, spread the mixture over the chicken and leave to marinate in a cool place for at least 20 minutes.

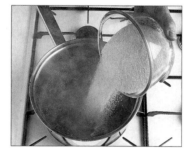

2 Meanwhile, bring the chicken stock to the boil in a heavy-based saucepan. Add the polenta in a steady stream, stirring all the time until thick: this will take 2–3 minutes. Turn out the cooked polenta on to a 2.5cm/1in-deep buttered tray and allow to cool.

COOK'S TIP

Lavender marinade is an unusual and quite delicious flavouring that goes well with saltwater fish as well as chicken. Try it, for example, over grilled cod, haddock, halibut, sea bass and bream.

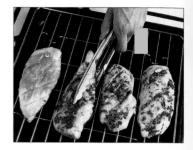

3 Heat the grill to moderate. Grill the chicken for about 15 minutes, turning once.

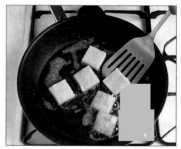

4 Cut the polenta into 2.5cm/1in cubes with a wet knife. Heat the butter in a large frying pan and fry the polenta cubes until golden.

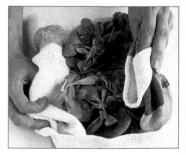

5 Wash the salad leaves and pat dry, then divide among 6 serving plates. Slice each chicken breast and lay over the salad. Place the polenta among the salad, decorate with the lavender and tomatoes, season and serve.

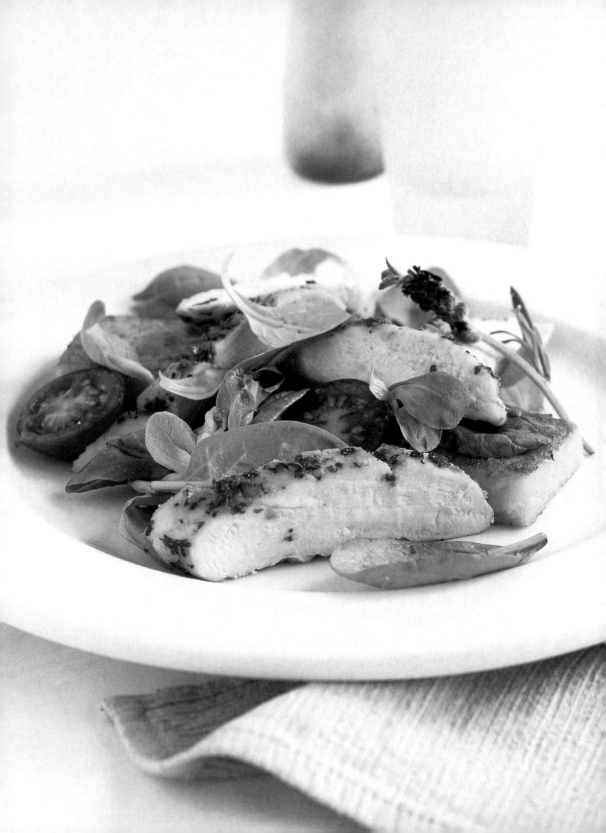

Tuna Carpaccio

Beef is usual for this Italian dish, but tuna makes a nice change.

INGREDIENTS

Serves 4

2 fresh tuna steaks, weighing 450g/1lb
   in total
60ml/4 tbsp extra virgin olive oil
15ml/1 tbsp balsamic vinegar
5ml/1 tsp caster sugar
30ml/2 tbsp drained bottled green
   peppercorns or capers
salt and freshly ground black pepper
lemon wedges and green salad, to serve

NUTRITION NOTES

Per portion:

Energy	257Kcals/1075kJ
Fat, total	16.2g
saturated fat	2.9g
Protein	26.6g
Carbohydrate	1.5g
sugar, total	1.5g
Fibre – NSP	0g
Sodium	53mg

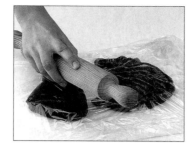

1 Remove the skin from each tuna steak and place each steak between two sheets of clear film or greaseproof paper. Pound with a rolling pin until slightly flattened.

COOK'S TIP

Raw fish is safe to eat as long as it is very fresh, so check with your fishmonger before purchasing, and make and serve the carpaccio on the same day. Do not buy fish that has been frozen and thawed.

2 Roll up the tuna as tightly as possible, then wrap tightly in clear film and place in the freezer for 4 hours or until firm.

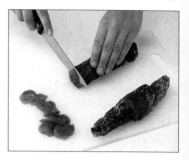

3 Unwrap the tuna and cut crossways into the thinnest slices possible. Arrange on individual plates.

4 Whisk together the remaining ingredients, season and pour over the tuna. Cover and allow to reach room temperature – this should take about 30 minutes – before serving with lemon wedges and green salad.

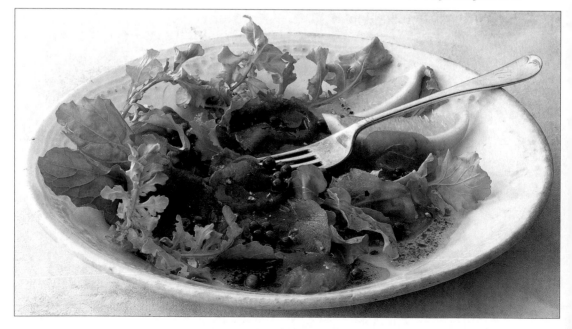

Baked Sweet Potato Salad

Sweet potato is cooked without any fat or oil, and the dressing is yogurt-based. What could be healthier or more delicious?

INGREDIENTS

Serves 4
900g/2lb sweet potatoes

For the dressing
45ml/3 tbsp chopped fresh coriander
juice of 1 lime
150ml/¼ pint/⅔ cup natural yogurt

For the salad
1 red pepper, seeded, finely chopped
3 celery sticks, finely chopped
¼ red onion, finely chopped
1 red chilli, finely chopped
salt and freshly ground black pepper
fresh coriander leaves, to garnish

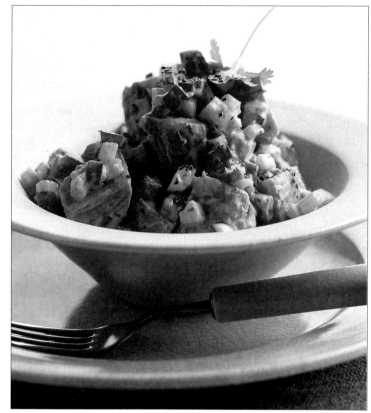

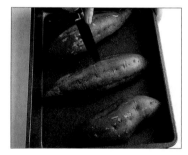

1 Preheat the oven to 200°C/400°F/ Gas 6. Wash and pierce the potatoes all over and bake in the oven for 40 minutes or until tender.

2 Meanwhile, mix the dressing ingredients together in a bowl and season to taste. Chill while you prepare the remaining ingredients.

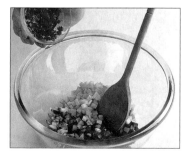

3 In a large bowl mix together the red pepper, celery, onion and chilli.

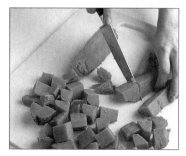

4 Remove the potatoes from the oven and, when cool enough to handle, peel them. Cut the potatoes into cubes and add them to the bowl. Drizzle the dressing over and toss carefully. Season again to taste and serve, garnished with fresh coriander.

— NUTRITION NOTES —	
Per portion:	
Energy	236Kcals/987kJ
Fat, total	1.2g
saturated fat	0.4g
Protein	5.3g
Carbohydrate	54.7g
sugar, total	19.2g
Fibre – NSP	6.5g
Sodium	136mg

Vegetable and Pasta Salad

Tender young vegetables in a light dressing make a delicious lunch. The vibrant colours and crunchy texture of the vegetables make this salad irresistible.

INGREDIENTS

Serves 4

225g/8oz/2 cups dried pasta shapes
115g/4oz baby carrots, trimmed and halved
115g/4oz baby sweetcorn, halved lengthways
50g/2oz mangetouts
115g/4oz young asparagus spears, trimmed
4 spring onions, trimmed and shredded
10ml/2 tsp white wine vinegar
60ml/4 tbsp extra virgin olive oil
15ml/1 tbsp wholegrain mustard
salt and freshly ground black pepper

1 Bring a large pan of salted water to the boil. Add the pasta and cook for 10–12 minutes, until just tender. Meanwhile, cook the carrots and sweetcorn in a second pan of boiling salted water for 5 minutes.

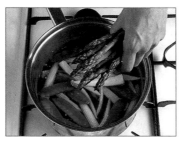

2 Add the mangetouts and asparagus to the carrot mixture and cook for 2–3 minutes. Drain the vegetables, refresh under cold water, drain again.

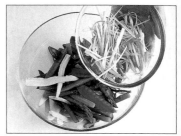

3 Tip the vegetable mixture into a mixing bowl, add the spring onions and toss well together.

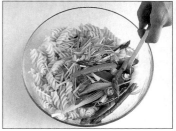

4 Drain the pasta, refresh it under cold running water and drain again. Toss with the vegetables.

5 Mix the vinegar, olive oil and mustard in a jar. Add salt and pepper to taste, close the jar tightly and shake well. Pour the dressing over the salad. Toss well and serve.

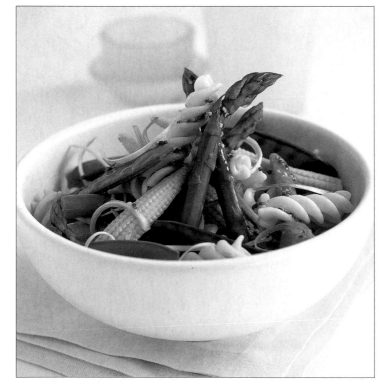

NUTRITION NOTES	
Per portion:	
Energy	492Kcals/2061kJ
Fat, total	18.9g
saturated fat	2.7g
Protein	14.1g
Carbohydrate	69.9g
sugar, total	7.2g
Fibre – NSP	6.1g
Sodium	138mg

Potato and Mixed Vegetable Salad

This chunky salad makes a satisfying meal. Use other spring vegetables, if you like.

INGREDIENTS

Serves 4

675g/1½lb small new potatoes, halved
400g/14oz can broad beans, drained
115g/4oz cherry tomatoes
50g/2oz/½ cup walnut halves
30ml/2 tbsp white wine vinegar
15ml/1 tbsp wholegrain mustard
60ml/4 tbsp olive oil
pinch of sugar
225g/8oz young asparagus
  spears, trimmed
6 spring onions, trimmed
salt and freshly ground black pepper
baby spinach leaves, to serve

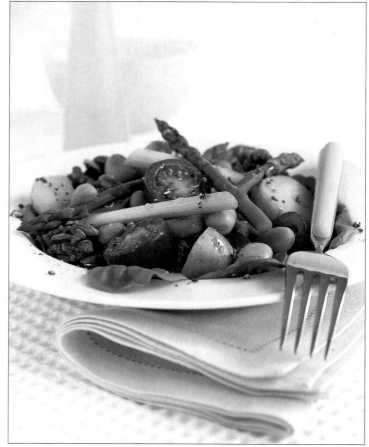

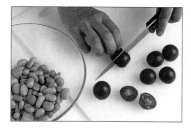

1 Put the potatoes in a pan. Cover with cold water and bring to the boil. Cook for 10–12 minutes until tender. Meanwhile, put the broad beans in a bowl. Cut the tomatoes in half and add them to the bowl with the walnuts.

2 Put the white wine vinegar, mustard, olive oil and sugar into a bowl. Add salt and pepper to taste. Whisk the dressing to mix well.

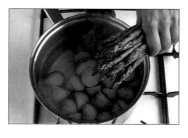

3 Add the asparagus to the potatoes and cook for 3 minutes more. Drain the cooked vegetables well, cool under cold running water and drain again. Thickly slice the potatoes. Cut the spring onions in half.

4 Add asparagus, potatoes and spring onions to the bean mixture. Toss in the dressing and serve with spinach.

NUTRITION NOTES	
Per portion:	
Energy	417Kcals/1744kJ
Fat, total	21.6g
saturated fat	2.6g
Protein	15.4g
Carbohydrate	42.8g
sugar, total	5.6g
Fibre – NSP	8.6g
Sodium	371mg

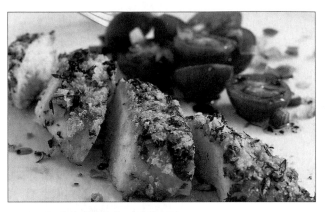

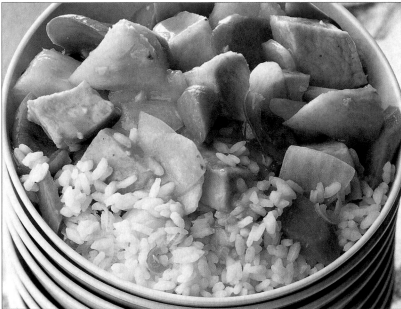

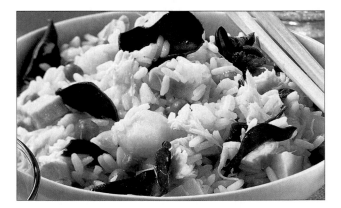

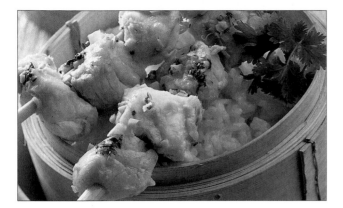

MEAT, POULTRY
AND SEAFOOD

Be it meat, poultry or seafood, the main course of any meal is its

pièce de résistance. Choose from this varied repertoire of tempting

dishes from round the world, such as Sweet-and-Sour Pork, Chicken

with Cashew Nuts, Monkfish and Scallop Skewers or Sea Bass en

Papillotte, and rest assured that your choice was a wise one and

as healthy as it was delicious.

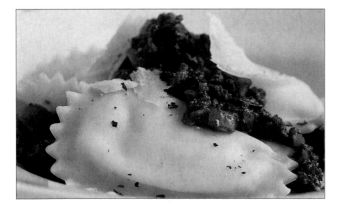

Marinated Lamb Kebabs

This modern version of the kebab uses marinated ultra-lean lamb, which is then grilled with chunks of vegetables. A delicious, healthy meal served with rice.

INGREDIENTS

Serves 6

500g/1¼lb lean lamb, cut into 4cm/
   1½in cubes
12 shallots or button onions
2 green peppers, seeded and cut into
   12 pieces
12 small tomatoes
12 small mushrooms
lemon slices and sprigs of rosemary,
   to garnish

For the marinade
juice of 1 lemon
120ml/4fl oz/½ cup red wine
1 onion, finely chopped
60ml/4 tbsp olive oil
2.5ml/½ tsp each dried sage
   and rosemary
salt and freshly ground black pepper

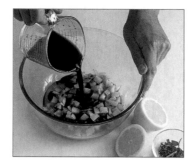

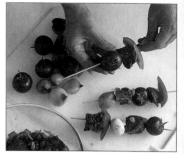

1 To make the marinade, combine the lemon juice, red wine, shallots or button onions, olive oil, herbs and seasoning in a bowl.

2 Stir the cubes of lamb into the marinade, mixing well. Cover and chill for about 2–3 hours, or longer if possible, stirring occasionally.

COOK'S TIP

For a vegetarian option, use cubes of tofu (beancurd) instead of the lamb.

---

3 Remove the lamb cubes from the marinade and thread on to six skewers with the shallots or onions, peppers, tomatoes and mushrooms.

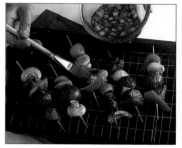

4 Cook the kebabs over the barbecue or under a preheated grill for 10–15 minutes, turning them once. Use the leftover marinade to brush over the kebabs during cooking to prevent the meat drying out.

5 Serve the kebabs garnished with sprigs of rosemary and lemon slices.

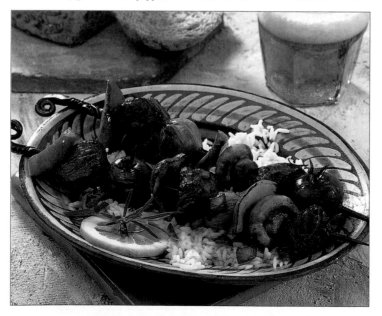

NUTRITION NOTES

Per portion:

Energy	232Kcals/970kJ
Fat, total	14.6g
saturated fat	4.3g
Protein	18.2g
Carbohydrate	4g
sugar, total	3.6g
Fibre – NSP	1.8g
Sodium	69mg

Spicy Meatballs with Red Rice

The flavours of fresh parsley, coriander and mint meld with ground cumin, cinnamon and ginger to create a wonderfully aromatic dish for which the nutty flavour of this interesting red rice is the perfect foil.

INGREDIENTS

Serves 6

225g/8oz/generous 1 cup Camargue
   red rice
675g/1½lb lamb leg steaks
2 onions
3–4 fresh parsley sprigs
3 fresh coriander sprigs, plus 30ml/
   2 tbsp chopped fresh coriander
1–2 fresh mint sprigs
2.5ml/½ tsp ground cumin
2.5ml/½ tsp ground cinnamon
2.5ml/½ tsp ground ginger
5ml/1 tsp paprika
30ml/2 tbsp sunflower oil
1 garlic clove, crushed
300ml/½ pint/1¼ cups tomato juice
450ml/¾ pint/scant 2 cups chicken
   or vegetable stock
salt and freshly ground black pepper

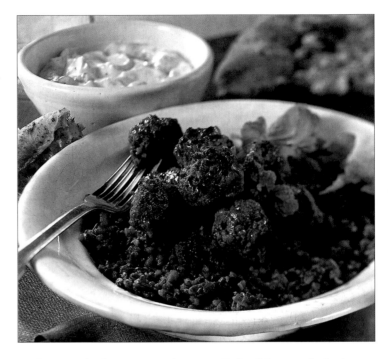

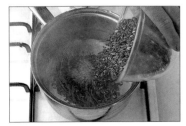

1 Cook the rice in plenty of lightly salted water or stock for 30 minutes or according to the instructions on the packet. Drain.

2 Meanwhile, prepare the meatballs. Chop the lamb roughly, then place it in a food processor and process until finely chopped. Scrape the meat into a large bowl.

3 Cut one onion into quarters and place in the processor with the parsley, coriander and mint sprigs; process until finely chopped. Return the lamb to the processor, add the spices and seasoning and process again until smooth. Scrape the mixture into a bowl and chill for about 1 hour.

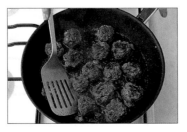

4 Shape the mixture into about 30 small balls. Heat half the oil in a frying pan, add the meatballs, in batches if necessary, and brown them evenly. Transfer to a plate. Chop the remaining onion finely.

5 Drain off the excess fat, leaving around 30ml/2 tbsp in the pan, and fry the chopped onion with the garlic for a few minutes until softened. Stir in the rice. Cook, stirring for 1–2 minutes, then stir in the tomato juice, stock and chopped fresh coriander. Season to taste with salt and pepper.

6 Arrange the meatballs over the rice, cover with a lid or foil and simmer gently for 15 minutes before serving.

NUTRITION NOTES	
Per portion:	
Energy	402Kcals/1681kJ
Fat, total	18.3g
saturated fat	7g
Protein	25.9g
Carbohydrate	33.4g
sugar, total	3.7g
Fibre – NSP	0.9g
Sodium	423mg

Beef Teriyaki

Lean beef prepared with a ginger and garlic marinade is simply grilled to make a healthy and delicious meal, served with a garnish of mooli and sprigs of fresh coriander.

INGREDIENTS

Serves 4

15ml/1 tbsp oil
60ml/4 tbsp soy sauce
30ml/2 tbsp mirin or medium sherry
5ml/1 tsp soft light brown sugar
15ml/1 tbsp ginger juice
  (see Cook's Tip)
1 garlic clove, crushed
500g/1¼lb rump steak, about
  2.5cm/1in thick, in one piece
  if possible
sansho pepper
1 mooli, peeled
30ml/2 tbsp wasabi paste and fresh
  coriander sprigs, to garnish

1 Mix the oil, soy sauce, mirin or sherry, sugar, ginger juice and garlic in a large shallow dish. Add the steak and turn to coat both sides. Leave in a cool place to marinate for at least 4 hours, turning from time to time.

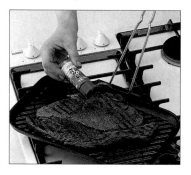

2 Preheat a grill, ridged cast-iron grill pan or barbecue, and grill the steak for 3–5 minutes on each side. Season with sansho pepper.

3 To prepare the Japanese-style garnish, grate the mooli and squeeze out as much liquid as possible. Place a little pile of grated mooli, with 7.5ml/1½ tsp of wasabi paste and a coriander sprig on each of four plates.

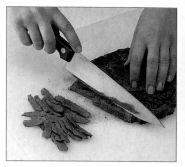

4 With a sharp knife, slice the steak into thin diagonal slices and arrange on the plates with the garnish.

COOK'S TIP

To make ginger juice, peel and grate a knob of fresh root ginger and squeeze out the liquid.

NUTRITION NOTES

Per portion:

Energy	207Kcals/866kJ
Fat, total	7.9g
saturated fat	2.5g
Protein	28.5g
Carbohydrate	3.6g
sugar, total	2.4g
Fibre – NSP	0g
Sodium	85mg

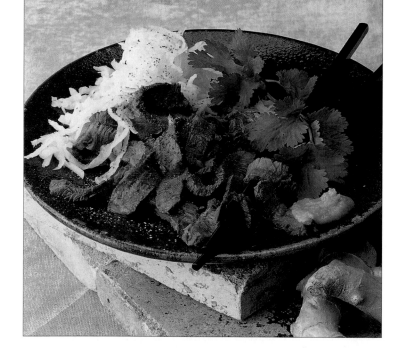

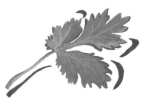

Ravioli with Bolognese Sauce

Make sure you buy the best quality minced beef for this dish. Then you can be sure that it has a low fat content.

INGREDIENTS

Serves 6
For the pasta dough
200g/7oz/1¾ cups plain four
pinch of salt
2 eggs
10ml/2 tsp cold water

For the filling
225g/8oz low-fat ricotta cheese
30ml/2 tbsp grated Parmesan cheese,
  plus extra to serve
1 egg white, beaten
1.5ml/¼ tsp grated nutmeg
1 onion, finely chopped
1 garlic clove, crushed
150ml/¼ pint/⅔ cup beef stock
350g/12oz extra-lean minced beef
120ml/4fl oz/½ cup red wine
30ml/2 tbsp tomato purée
400g/14oz can chopped tomatoes
2.5ml/½ tsp chopped fresh rosemary
1.5ml/¼ tsp ground allspice
salt and freshly ground black pepper

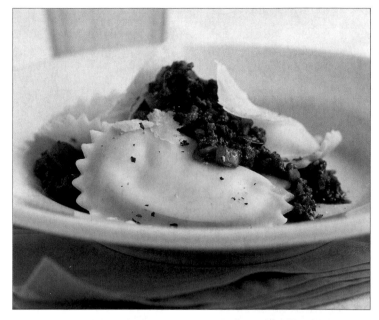

1 To make the pasta, sift the flour and salt on to a work surface and make a well. Put the eggs and water into the well. Beat the eggs together, then draw in the flour from the sides, to make a thick paste. Mix to a firm dough, then knead until smooth. Wrap in clear film and leave to rest for 20–30 minutes.

2 To make the filling, mix together the ricotta cheese, Parmesan, egg white, seasoning and grated nutmeg.

3 Roll the pasta into thin sheets, place a small teaspoonful of filling along the pasta in rows 5cm/2in apart. Moisten the pasta between the filling with beaten egg white. Lay a second sheet of pasta lightly over the top and press between each pocket to remove any air and seal firmly.

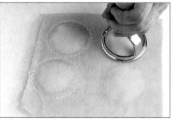

4 Cut into rounds with a serrated ravioli or pastry cutter. Transfer to a floured cloth and rest for at least 30 minutes before cooking.

NUTRITION NOTES	
Per portion:	
Energy	340Kcals/1422kJ
Fat, total	11.7g
saturated fat	5.7g
Protein	23.5g
Carbohydrate	33.1g
sugar, total	5.4g
Fibre – NSP	2g
Sodium	298mg

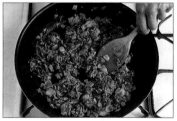

5 To make the Bolognese sauce, cook the onion and garlic in the stock for 5 minutes or until the stock has reduced. Add the beef and cook quickly to brown, breaking it up with a spoon. Add the wine, tomato purée, chopped tomatoes, rosemary and allspice, bring to the boil and simmer for 1 hour. Adjust the seasoning.

6 Cook the ravioli in a large pan of boiling, salted water for about 4-5 minutes. (Cook in batches to stop them sticking together.) Drain thoroughly. Serve topped with Bolognese sauce, and hand round grated Parmesan cheese separately.

Sweet-and-sour Pork

In this wonderful low-fat version of a popular, classic Chinese stir-fry dish, the flavours are not compromised at all.

INGREDIENTS

Serves 4

15ml/1 tbsp dry sherry
350g/12oz lean pork steaks
15ml/1 tbsp vegetable oil
1 garlic clove, finely chopped
½ onion, diced
1 small green pepper, seeded and cut
   into 2.5cm/1in squares
1 small carrot, sliced
75g/3oz/½ cup drained, canned
   pineapple chunks
30ml/2 tbsp malt vinegar
45ml/3 tbsp tomato ketchup
150ml/¼ pint/⅔ cup pineapple juice
2.5ml/½ tsp caster sugar
2.5ml/½ tsp cornflour
15ml/1 tbsp cold water
salt and freshly ground black pepper
rice, steamed or fried, to serve

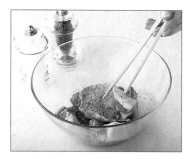

1 Mix the sherry, 2.5ml/½ tsp salt and a large pinch of pepper in a large bowl or shallow dish. Add the pork, turn well to coat thoroughly, then cover and leave to marinate in a cool place for 15 minutes.

COOK'S TIP

If you prefer, this dish is equally delicious served with noodles instead of rice.

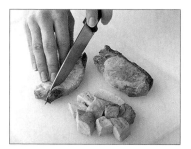

2 Drain the pork steaks and place them on a rack over a grill pan. Grill under a high heat for 5 minutes on each side or until cooked, then remove and leave to cool. Cut the cooked pork into bite-size pieces, trimming off any bits of fat.

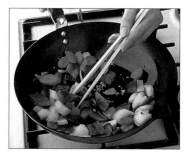

3 Heat the oil in a non-stick frying pan or wok until very hot. Stir-fry the garlic and onion for a few seconds, then add the green pepper and carrot and stir-fry for 1 minute more.

--- NUTRITION NOTES ---

Per portion:

Energy	185Kcals/744kJ
Fat, total	6.2g
saturated fat	0.4g
Protein	20g
Carbohydrate	12.2g
sugar, total	11.6g
Fibre – NSP	1.2g
Sodium	194mg

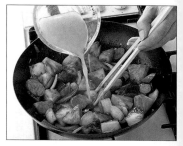

4 Stir in the pineapple chunks, vinegar, tomato ketchup, pineapple juice and caster sugar. Quickly bring to the boil, lower the heat and simmer for 3 minutes.

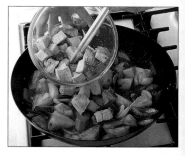

5 Add the pieces of cooked pork to the vegetable mixture, stir well and cook for about 2 minutes.

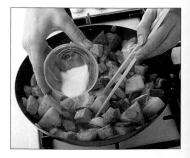

6 In a small bowl, mix the cornflour to a paste with the water. Add the mixture to the pan or wok and cook, stirring, until slightly thickened. Serve with rice, either steamed or fried as you prefer.

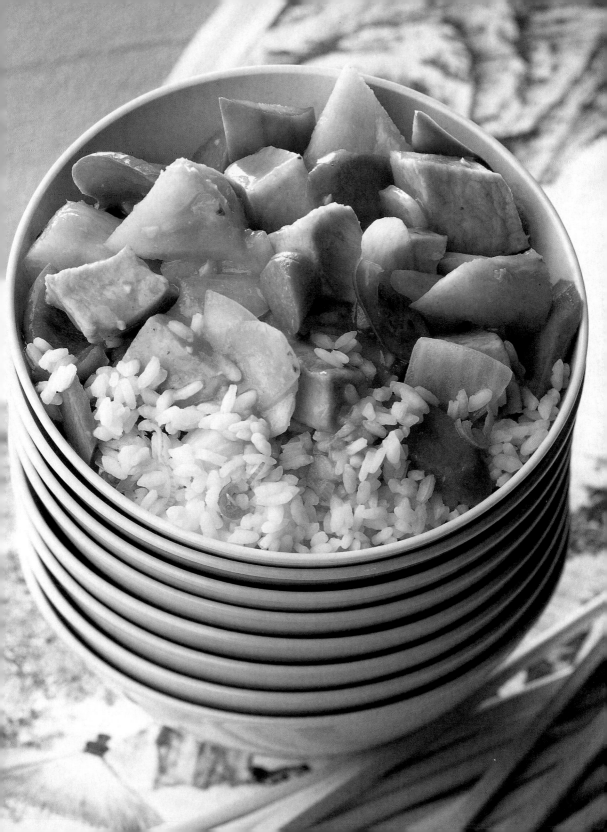

Chicken with Cashew Nuts

Stir-frying is a really healthy way of preparing food. It uses just the minimum of oil, and the mix of vegetables cooked by this method remain crunchy and fresh.

Ingredients

Serves 4
350g/12oz skinless chicken
   breast fillets
1.5ml/¼ tsp salt
pinch of ground white pepper
15ml/1 tbsp dry sherry
300ml/½ pint/1¼ cups chicken stock
15ml/1 tbsp vegetable oil
1 garlic clove, finely chopped
1 small carrot, cut into cubes
½ cucumber, about 75g/3oz, cut into
   1cm/½ in cubes
50g/2oz/½ cup drained canned
   bamboo shoots, cut into
   1cm/½in cubes
5ml/1 tsp cornflour
15ml/1 tbsp light soy sauce
5ml/1 tsp caster sugar
25g/1oz/¼ cup dry roasted cashew nuts
2.5ml/½ tsp sesame oil
noodles, to serve

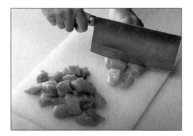

1 Cut the chicken breast fillets into 2cm/¾in cubes. Place the chicken cubes in a bowl, stir in the salt, pepper and sherry, cover and marinate for at least 15 minutes.

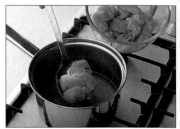

2 Bring the stock to the boil in a large saucepan. Add the chicken and cook, stirring, for 3 minutes. Drain, reserving 90ml/6 tbsp of the stock, and set aside.

— Nutrition Notes —	
Per portion:	
Energy	174Kcals/728kJ
Fat, total	6.9g
saturated fat	1.2g
Protein	23.9g
Carbohydrate	2.9g
sugar, total	1.5g
Fibre – NSP	0.9g
Sodium	421mg

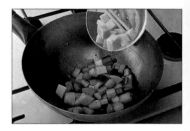

3 Heat the vegetable oil in a non-stick frying pan until very hot, add the garlic and stir-fry for a few seconds. Add the carrot, cucumber and bamboo shoots, and continue to stir-fry over a medium heat for 2 minutes.

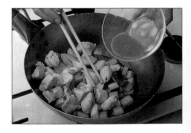

4 Stir in the chicken and reserved stock. Mix the cornflour with the soy sauce and sugar, and add the mixture to the pan. Cook, stirring, until the sauce thickens slightly. Finally, add the cashew nuts and sesame oil. Toss to mix thoroughly then serve with noodles.

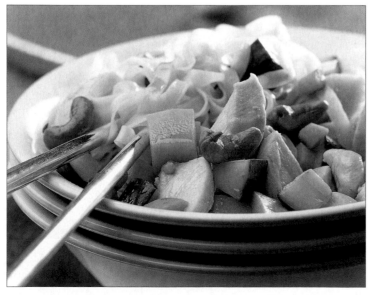

Pasta Bows with Chicken and Cherry Tomatoes

Quick to prepare and easy to cook, this colourful dish is full of flavour. For an even healthier option, omit the salami.

INGREDIENTS

Serves 6

350g/12oz skinless chicken breast
  fillets, cut into bite-size pieces
60ml/4 tbsp Italian dry vermouth
10ml/2 tsp chopped fresh rosemary,
  plus 4 fresh rosemary sprigs,
  to garnish
15ml/1 tbsp olive oil
1 onion, finely chopped
90g/3½oz piece Italian salami, diced
275g/10oz/2½ cups dried pasta bows
15ml/1 tbsp balsamic vinegar
400g/14oz can Italian cherry tomatoes
good pinch of crushed dried red chillies
salt and freshly ground black pepper

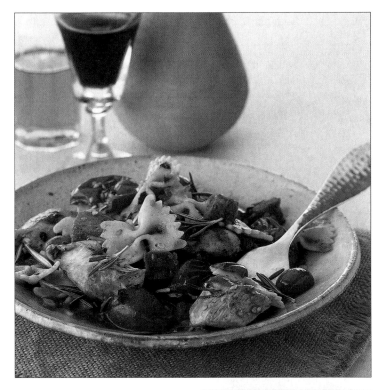

1 Put the pieces of chicken in a large bowl, pour in the dry vermouth and sprinkle with half the chopped rosemary and salt and pepper to taste. Stir well and set aside.

2 Heat the oil in a large skillet or saucepan, add the onion and salami and fry over a medium heat for about 5 minutes, stirring frequently,

3 Cook the pasta according to the instructions on the packet.

NUTRITION NOTES	
Per portion:	
Energy	334Kcals/1397kJ
Fat, total	9.2g
saturated fat	2.8g
Protein	23.6g
Carbohydrate	39g
sugar, total	4.6g
Fibre – NSP	2.2g
Sodium	337mg

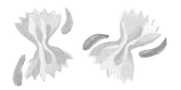

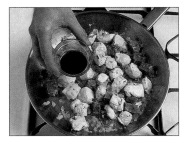

4 Add the chicken and vermouth to the onion and salami, increase the heat to high and fry for 3 minutes or until the chicken is white on all sides. Sprinkle the vinegar over the chicken.

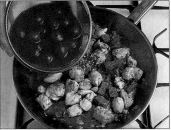

5 Add the cherry tomatoes and dried chillies. Stir well and simmer for a few minutes more. Taste the sauce and adjust the seasoning if necessary.

6 Drain the pasta and tip it into the skillet or saucepan. Add the remaining chopped rosemary and toss to mix the pasta and sauce together. Serve immediately in warmed bowls, garnished with the rosemary sprigs.

Chicken in Herb Crusts

Chicken is always a good option for those who are watching their weight. These lovely herbed crusts are guaranteed to make your mouth water.

INGREDIENTS

Serves 4
4 boned and skinned chicken breasts
15ml/1 tbsp Dijon mustard
30ml/2 tbsp chopped fresh parsley
50g/2oz/1 cup fresh breadcrumbs
15ml/1 tbsp dried mixed herbs
25g/1oz/2 tbsp butter, melted
salt and freshly ground black pepper

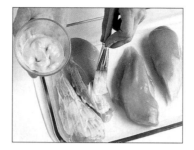

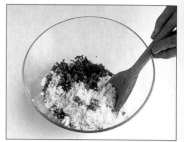

1 Preheat the oven to 180°C/350°F/ Gas 4. Lay the chicken in a greased ovenproof dish and spread with the mustard. Season with salt and pepper.

2 In a large bowl, mix the fresh parsley, breadcrumbs and the dried mixed herbs together thoroughly.

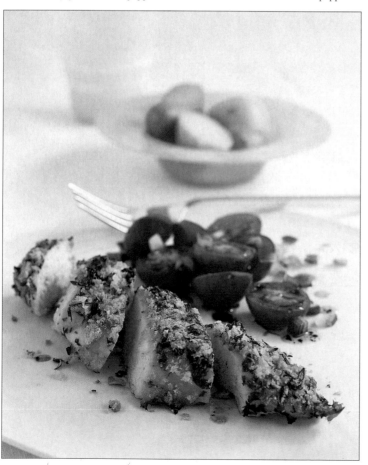

3 Press on to the chicken to coat. Spoon over the melted butter. Bake uncovered for 20 minutes or until tender and crisp.

COOK'S TIP

The chicken breasts can be brushed with melted butter instead of mustard before being coated in the breadcrumb mixture.

NUTRITION NOTES

Per portion:

Energy	254Kcals/1062kJ
Fat, total	7.3g
saturated fat	3.9g
Protein	37.7g
Carbohydrate	10.1g
sugar, total	0.6g
Fibre – NSP	0.3g
Sodium	342mg

Chicken Biryani

The intense flavours of this dish are nicely balanced by the fresh taste of the natural yogurt.

INGREDIENTS

Serves 4

10 whole green cardamom pods
275g/10oz/1½ cups basmati rice,
   soaked and drained
2.5ml/½ tsp salt
2–3 whole cloves
5cm/2in cinnamon stick
45ml/3 tbsp vegetable oil
3 onions, sliced
4 chicken breasts, each about
   175g/6oz, cubed
1.5ml/¼ tsp ground cloves
1.5ml/¼ tsp hot chilli powder
5ml/1 tsp ground cumin
5ml/1 tsp ground coriander
2.5ml/½ tsp ground black pepper
3 garlic cloves, chopped
5ml/1 tsp chopped fresh root ginger
juice of 1 lemon
4 tomatoes, sliced
30ml/2 tbsp chopped fresh coriander
150ml/¼ pint/⅔ cup natural yogurt,
   plus extra, to serve
4–5 saffron threads, soaked in 10ml/
   2 tsp hot milk
150ml/¼ pint/⅔ cup water
toasted flaked almonds and fresh
   coriander sprigs, to garnish

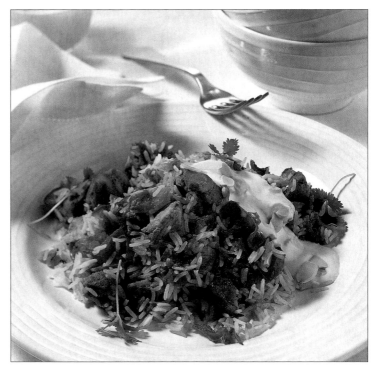

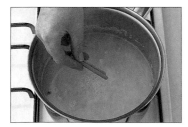

1 Preheat the oven to 190°C/375°F/ Gas 5. Deseed half the cardamom pods, grind the seeds and set aside. To a pan of boiling water, add the rice, salt, whole cardamom pods, cloves and cinnamon, and boil for 2 minutes. Drain, leaving the spices in the rice.

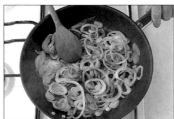

2 Heat the oil in a frying pan and fry the onions for 8 minutes, until softened and browned. Add the chicken and the ground spices, including the ground cardamom seeds. Mix well, then add the garlic, ginger and lemon juice. Stir-fry for 5 minutes.

3 Transfer the chicken mixture to a casserole and arrange the tomatoes on top. Sprinkle on the fresh coriander, spoon the yogurt evenly on top and cover with the drained rice.

4 Drizzle the saffron milk over the rice and pour over the water. Cover tightly and bake for 1 hour.

5 Transfer to a warmed serving platter and remove the whole spices from the rice. Garnish with toasted almonds and fresh coriander sprigs, and serve with the natural yogurt.

NUTRITION NOTES	
Per portion:	
Energy	376Kcals/1586kJ
Fat, total	7.4g
saturated fat	1.1g
Protein	33.6g
Carbohydrate	44.2g
sugar, total	6.44g
Fibre – NSP	1.2g
Sodium	97mg

PROPERTY OF
WALNUT PUBLIC
LIBRARY DISTRICT

Monkfish and Scallop Skewers

Lemon and coriander team up beautifully with the seafood in these chunky fish kebabs.

INGREDIENTS

Serves 4

450g/1lb monkfish fillet
8 lemon grass stalks
30ml/2 tbsp fresh lemon juice
15ml/1 tbsp olive oil
15ml/1 tbsp finely chopped
  fresh coriander
2.5ml/½ tsp salt
large pinch of ground black pepper
12 large scallops, halved crossways
a few fresh coriander leaves,
  to garnish
rice, to serve

<table>
<tr><td>—— VARIATION ——</td></tr>
<tr><td>Raw tiger prawns and salmon make excellent alternative ingredients for the skewers, with or without the monkfish.</td></tr>
</table>

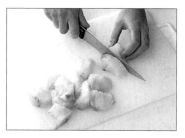

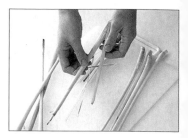

1 Remove any membrane from the monkfish, then cut into 16 chunks.

NUTRITION NOTES	
Per portion:	
Energy	158Kcals/661kJ
Fat, total	3.9g
saturated fat	0.7g
Protein	29.2g
Carbohydrate	1.7g
sugar, total	0g
Fibre – NSP	0g
Sodium	110mg

2 Remove the outer leaves from the lemon grass to leave thin rigid stalks. Chop the tender parts of the lemon grass leaves finely and place in a bowl. Stir in the lemon juice, oil, chopped coriander, salt and pepper.

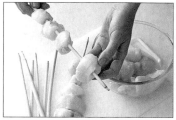

3 Thread the fish and scallop chunks alternately on to the eight lemon grass stalks. Arrange the skewers of fish and shellfish in a shallow dish and pour over the marinade.

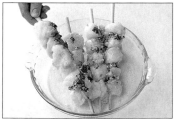

4 Cover and leave in a cool place for 1 hour, turning occasionally. Transfer the skewers to a heatproof dish or bamboo steamer, cover and steam over boiling water for 10 minutes until just cooked. Garnish with coriander and serve with rice and the cooking juice poured over.

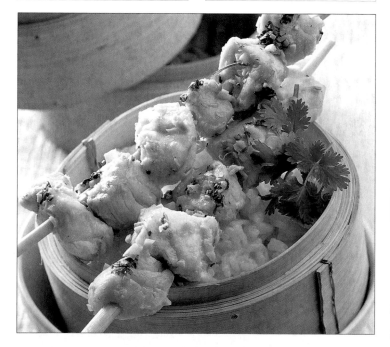

Seafood Conchiglie

This spicy warm salad of scallops, pasta and fresh rocket leaves will relieve anyone's hunger pangs and takes only minutes to prepare.

INGREDIENTS

Serves 4

8 large fresh scallops
300g/11oz/2¾ cups dried pasta shells
15ml/1 tbsp olive oil
15g/½oz/1 tbsp butter
120ml/4fl oz/½ cup dry white wine
90g/3½oz rocket leaves, stalks trimmed
salt and freshly ground black pepper

For the vinaigrette

60ml/4 tbsp extra virgin olive oil
15ml/1 tbsp balsamic vinegar
1 piece bottled roasted pepper, drained
 and finely chopped
1–2 fresh red chillies, seeded
 and chopped
1 garlic clove, crushed
5–10ml/1–2 tsp clear honey

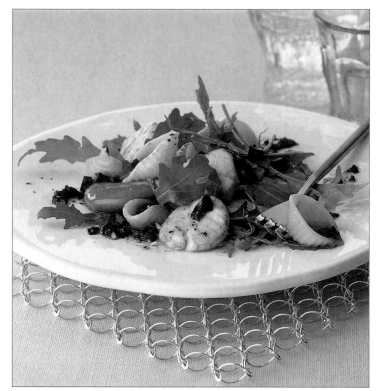

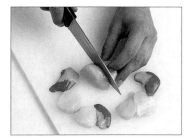

1 Cut each scallop into 2–3 pieces. If the corals are attached, pull them off and cut each piece in half. Season the scallops and corals well with salt and pepper.

2 To make the vinaigrette, put the oil, vinegar, chopped pepper and chillies in a jug with the garlic and honey to taste. Whisk well.

3 Cook the pasta shells according to the instructions on the packet until *al dente*.

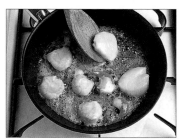

4 Meanwhile, heat the oil and butter in a frying pan until sizzling. Add half the scallops and toss over a high heat for 2 minutes. Remove with a slotted spoon and keep warm. Cook the remaining scallops in the same way.

5 Add the wine to the liquid in the pan and stir over a high heat until reduced to a few tablespoons.

6 Drain the pasta and tip it into a warmed bowl. Add the rocket, scallops, reduced cooking juices and vinaigrette, and toss well to combine all the ingredients. Serve immediately.

NUTRITION NOTES	
Per portion:	
Energy	500Kcals/2092kJ
Fat, total	19g
saturated fat	4.5g
Protein	20.3g
Carbohydrate	61.2g
sugar, total	4.5g
Fibre – NSP	3g
Sodium	150mg

Stir-fried Jewelled Rice

There are some wonderful contrasting textures and flavours in this jewel-like dish, from the delicate sweetness of crab meat to the vibrant crunch of the water chestnuts.

INGREDIENTS

Serves 4

350g/12oz/1¾ cups long grain rice
45ml/3 tbsp vegetable oil
1 onion, roughly chopped
4 dried black Chinese mushrooms,
  soaked for 10 minutes in warm water
  to cover
115g/4oz/⅔ cup cooked ham, diced
175g/6oz drained canned white
  crab meat
75g/3oz/½ cup drained canned
  water chestnuts
115g/4oz/1 cup peas, thawed if frozen
30ml/2 tbsp oyster sauce
5ml/1 tsp granulated sugar
salt

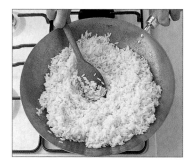

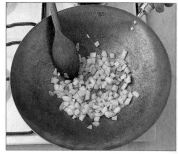

1 Rinse the rice and cook for 10–12 minutes in salted boiling water. Drain, refresh and drain again. Heat half the oil in a wok and, when hot, stir-fry the rice for 3 minutes. Set aside.

2 Heat the remaining oil in the wok and cook the onion until softened but not coloured. Drain the Chinese mushrooms, cut off and discard the stalks, then chop the caps.

COOK'S TIP

When adding oil to the hot wok, drizzle it in a "necklace" just below the rim. It will coat the inner surface as it heats.

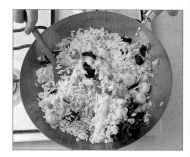

3 Add the chopped mushrooms to the wok, with all the remaining ingredients except the rice. Stir-fry for 2 minutes, then add the rice and stir-fry for about 3 minutes more. Serve at once.

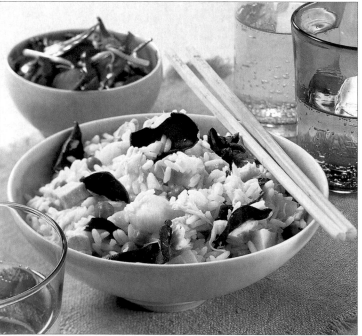

NUTRITION NOTES	
Per portion:	
Energy	525Kcals/2196kJ
Fat, total	13.4g
saturated fat	2.4g
Protein	22.9g
Carbohydrate	83.5g
sugar, total	3.6g
Fibre – NSP	2.3g
Sodium	862mg

Sea Bass en Papillote

By baking *en papillote*, all the aromas of the food are held within the package, intensifying the flavours. Bring the unopened packages to the table and let your guests open their own.

INGREDIENTS

Serves 4

4 small sea bass, gutted
115g/4oz/½ cup butter
450g/1lb spinach, washed well
3 shallots, finely chopped
60ml/4 tbsp white wine
4 bay leaves
salt and freshly ground black pepper

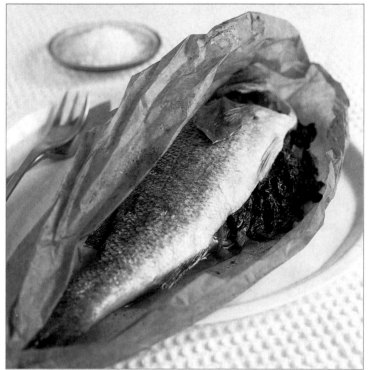

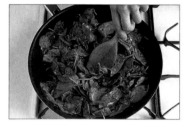

1 Preheat the oven to 180°C/350°F/ Gas 4. Season both the inside and outside of the fish. Melt 50g/2oz/ ¼ cup of the butter in a large, heavy-based frying pan and add the spinach. Cook gently until the spinach has broken down into a smooth purée. Set aside to cool.

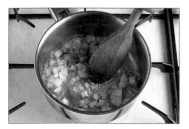

2 Melt the remainder of the butter in a clean pan and add the shallots. Gently sauté for 5 minutes until soft. Add to the spinach, season to taste with salt and black pepper, and leave to cool.

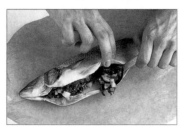

3 Using a tablespoon, stuff the insides of the fish with the spinach filling.

4 For each fish, fold a large sheet of greaseproof paper in half and cut around the fish to make a heart shape when the paper is unfolded. It should be at least 5cm/2in larger than the fish. Brush a little of the melted butter on to the paper. Set the fish on one side of the paper. Add a little wine and a bay leaf to each package.

5 Fold the other side of the paper over the fish and make small pleats to seal the two edges, starting at the curve of the heart shape. Brush the outsides of the paper with a little melted butter. Transfer the packages to a baking sheet and bake for 20–25 minutes until the packages are brown. Serve with baby vegetables.

NUTRITION NOTES	
Per portion:	
Energy	301Kcals/1259kJ
Fat, total	15.3g
saturated fat	7.6g
Protein	35.9g
Carbohydrate	2.5g
sugar, total	2.4g
Fibre – NSP	2.6g
Sodium	369mg

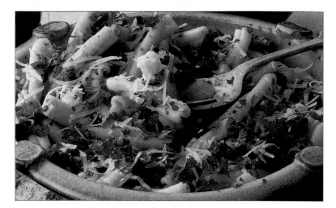

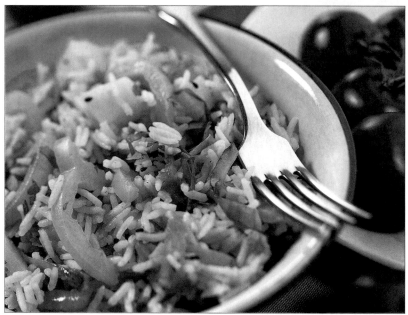

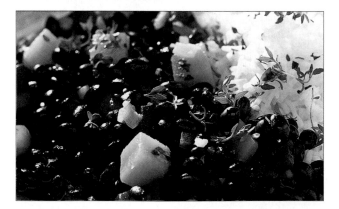

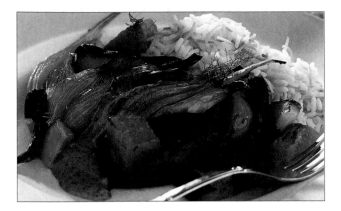

VEGETABLES, GRAINS AND PULSES

There is a great deal more versatility to these ingredients

than serving them as accompaniments to meat and fish.

Try, for example, Mixed Vegetable and New Potato Casserole,

Black Bean Hotpot, Broccoli, Chilli and Artichoke Pasta, or

Vegetable Couscous – all of which can be served as

delicious and satisfying main courses.

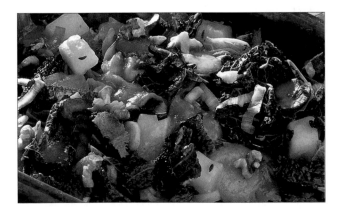

Spinach and Cannellini Beans

This tasty winter dish is warming without being too filling.

INGREDIENTS

Serves 4

225g/8oz/1¼ cups cannellini beans, soaked overnight
60ml/4 tbsp olive oil
1 slice white bread
1 onion, chopped
3–4 tomatoes, peeled and chopped
good pinch of paprika
450g/1lb spinach
1 garlic clove, halved
salt and freshly ground black pepper

1 Drain the beans, place in a saucepan and cover with water. Bring to the boil and fast boil for 10 minutes. Cover and simmer for 1 hour until the beans are tender. Drain.

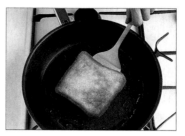

2 Heat 30ml/2 tbsp of the olive oil in a frying pan and fry the slice of bread until it is golden brown. Transfer to a plate.

3 Fry the chopped onion in 15ml/ 1 tbsp of the oil over a gentle heat until soft but not brown, then add the tomatoes and continue cooking over a gentle heat until the tomatoes are soft and cooked through.

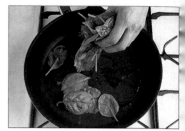

4 Heat the remaining oil in a pan, stir in the paprika and then add the spinach. Cover and cook for a few minutes until the spinach has wilted.

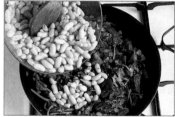

5 Add the onion and tomato mixture to the spinach, mix well and stir in the cannellini beans. Place the garlic and fried bread in a food processor and process until smooth.

6 Stir the processed garlic and bread into the spinach and bean mixture. Season with a little salt and black pepper, add 150ml/¼ pint/⅔ cup cold water, then cover and simmer gently for 20-30 minutes, adding more water if necessary.

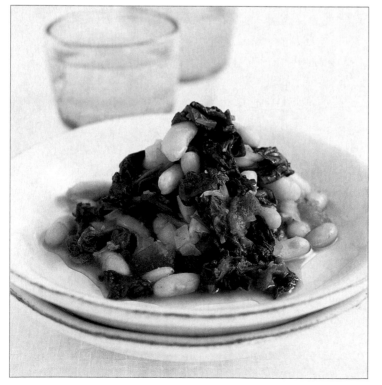

NUTRITION NOTES	
Per portion:	
Energy	331Kcals/1384kJ
Fat, total	13.1g
saturated fat	1.9g
Protein	16.7g
Carbohydrate	38.7g
sugar, total	7.2g
Fibre – NSP	13.1g
Sodium	234mg

Mixed Vegetable and New Potato Casserole

Here is a meal in a pot that's suitable for feeding large numbers of people. It's lightly spiced and the presence of garlic gives extra flavour without the addition of extra fat.

INGREDIENTS

Serves 4

60ml/4 tbsp olive oil
1 large onion, chopped
2 aubergines, cut into small cubes
4 courgettes, cut into small chunks
1 green pepper, seeded and chopped
1 red or yellow pepper, seeded
   and chopped
115g/4oz/1 cup fresh or frozen peas
115g/4oz French beans
450g/1lb new or salad potatoes, cubed
2.5ml/½ tsp cinnamon
2.5ml/½ tsp ground cumin
5ml/1 tsp paprika
4–5 tomatoes, skinned
400g/14oz can chopped tomatoes
30ml/2 tbsp chopped fresh parsley
3–4 garlic cloves, crushed
350ml/12fl oz/1½ cups vegetable stock
salt and freshly ground black pepper
black olives and chopped fresh parsley,
   to garnish

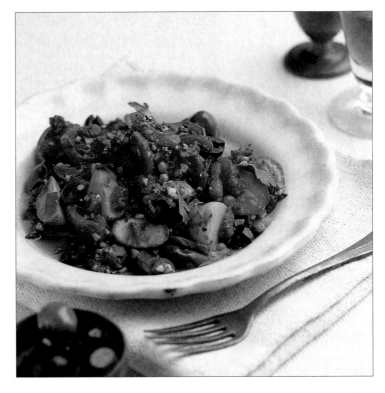

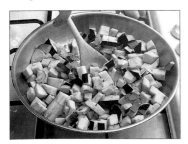

1 Preheat the oven to 190°C/375°F/ Gas 5. Heat 45ml/3 tbsp of the oil in a heavy-based pan, add the chopped onion and fry until golden then add the aubergines and sauté for 3 minutes. Add the courgettes, the green and the red or yellow peppers, peas, beans and potatoes, together with the spices and the salt and pepper. Stir well.

2 Continue to cook for 3 minutes, stirring all the time. Transfer to a shallow ovenproof dish.

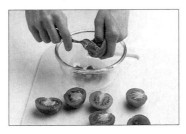

3 Halve, seed and chop the fresh tomatoes and mix with the canned tomatoes, parsley, garlic and the remaining olive oil in a bowl.

4 Pour the stock over the aubergine mixture and then spoon over the tomato mixture.

5 Bake for 30–45 minutes or until the vegetables are tender. Serve garnished with black olives and parsley.

COOK'S TIP

Omit the black olives from the garnish for this dish if you wish.

NUTRITION NOTES

Per portion:

Energy	307Kcals/1284kJ
Fat, total	13.2g
saturated fat	2.1g
Protein	10.3g
Carbohydrate	39.3g
sugar, total	18.2g
Fibre – NSP	9.3g
Sodium	247mg

Roasted Vegetables with Salsa Verde

Instead of a heavy, calorie-laden sauce to accompany these roast vegetables, try this salsa verde. Mint and parsley are combined with mustard and lemon to create a great piquant flavour.

INGREDIENTS

Serves 4

3 courgettes, sliced lengthways
1 large fennel bulb, cut into wedges
450g/1lb butternut squash, cut into
   2cm/¾in chunks
12 shallots
2 red peppers, seeded and cut
   lengthways into thick slices
4 plum tomatoes, halved and seeded
45ml/3 tbsp olive oil
2 garlic cloves, crushed
5ml/1 tsp balsamic vinegar
salt and freshly ground black pepper

For the salsa verde

45ml/3 tbsp chopped fresh mint
90ml/6 tbsp chopped fresh flat
   leaf parsley
15ml/1 tbsp Dijon mustard
juice of ½ lemon
30ml/2 tbsp olive oil

For the rice

15ml/1 tbsp vegetable or olive oil
75g/3oz/¾ cup vermicelli, broken into
   short lengths
225g/8oz/generous 1 cup long
   grain rice
900ml/1½ pints/3¾ cups vegetable
   stock

NUTRITION NOTES

Per portion:

Energy	524Kcals/2192kJ
Fat, total	17.4g
saturated fat	2.7g
Protein	11.5g
Carbohydrate	84.6g
sugar, total	16.9g
Fibre – NSP	7.1g
Sodium	141mg

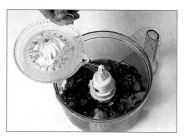

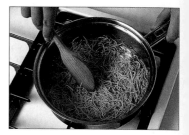

1 Preheat the oven to 220°C/425°F/ Gas 7. To make the salsa verde, place all the ingredients, with the exception of the olive oil, in a food processor or blender. Blend to a coarse paste, then add the oil, a little at a time, until the mixture forms a smooth purée. Season to taste.

2 To roast the vegetables, toss the courgettes, fennel, squash, shallots, peppers and tomatoes in the olive oil, garlic and balsamic vinegar. Leave for 10 minutes to allow all the flavours to mingle.

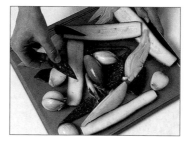

3 Place all the vegetables – apart from the squash and tomatoes – on a baking sheet, lightly brush with half the oil and vinegar mixture and season.

4 Roast for about 25 minutes, then remove the baking sheet from the oven. Turn the vegetables over and brush with the rest of the oil and vinegar mixture. Add the squash and plum tomatoes and cook for a further 20–25 minutes until all the vegetables are tender and lightly blackened around the edges.

5 Meanwhile, prepare the rice. Heat the oil in a heavy-based saucepan. Add the vermicelli and fry for about 3 minutes or until golden and crisp. Season to taste.

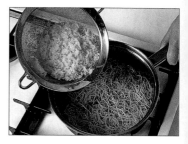

6 Rinse the rice under cold running water, then drain well and add it to the vermicelli. Cook for 1 minute, stirring to coat it in the oil.

7 Add the vegetable stock, then cover the pan and cook for about 12 minutes until the water is absorbed. Stir the rice, then cover and leave to stand for 10 minutes. Serve the warm rice with the roasted vegetables and salsa verde.

COOK'S TIP

The salsa verde will keep for up to 1 week if stored in an airtight container in the fridge.

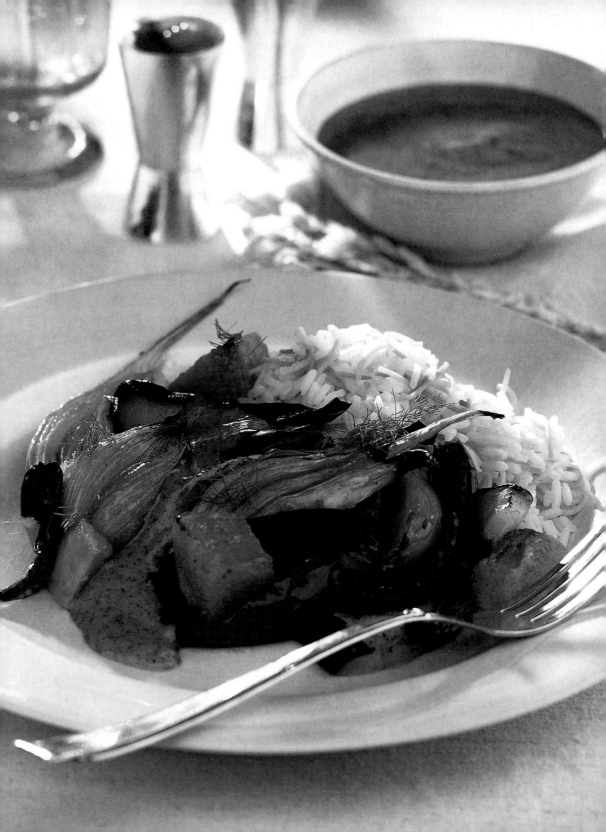

Curried Potatoes and Spinach

Traditional Indian spices, such as mustard seed, ginger, and chilli, give a really good kick to potatoes and spinach in this delicious and authentic curry, which could be served as a side dish or as a vegetarian main dish.

INGREDIENTS

Serves 4

450g/1lb spinach
30ml/2 tbsp vegetable oil
5ml/1 tsp black mustard seeds
1 onion, thinly sliced
2 garlic cloves, crushed
2.5cm/1in piece ginger root, finely chopped
675g/1½lb firm potatoes, cut into 2.5cm/1in chunks
5ml/1 tsp chilli powder
5ml/1 tsp salt
120ml/4fl oz/½ cup water

1 Blanch the spinach in boiling water for 3–4 minutes.

2 Drain the spinach thoroughly and leave to cool. When it is cool enough to handle, use your hands to squeeze out any remaining liquid, or roll it up in a dish towel and squeeze.

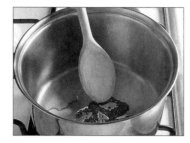

3 Heat the oil in a large saucepan and fry the mustard seeds for 2 minutes, stirring, until they begin to splutter.

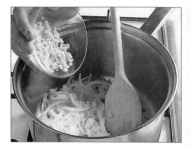

4 Add the onion, garlic and ginger, and fry for 5 minutes, stirring.

5 Stir in the potatoes, chilli powder, salt and water, and cook for 8 minutes, stirring occasionally.

6 Finally, add the spinach to the pan. Cover and simmer for 10–15 minutes until the spinach is cooked and the potatoes are tender. Serve hot.

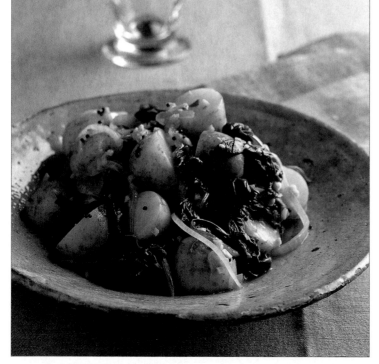

—— COOK'S TIP ——

Choose a firm, waxy variety of potato or a salad potato so the pieces do not break up during cooking.

—— NUTRITION NOTES ——

Per portion:

Energy	209Kcals/874kJ
Fat, total	6.9g
saturated fat	0.9g
Protein	6.4g
Carbohydrate	31.9g
sugar, total	5.9g
Fibre – NSP	4.6g
Sodium	668mg

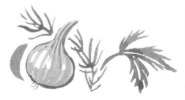

Black Bean Hotpot

Blackstrap molasses imparts a rich treacly flavour to the spicy sauce in this dish, as well as being beneficial to your general health. This dish incorporates a stunning mixture of black beans, peppers and squash or pumpkin and is delicious served with rice.

INGREDIENTS

Serves 4
225g/8oz/1¼ cups dried black beans
1 bay leaf
30ml/2 tbsp vegetable oil
1 large onion, chopped
1 garlic clove, chopped
5ml/1 tsp mustard powder
15ml/1 tbsp blackstrap molasses
30ml/2 tbsp soft dark brown sugar
5ml/1 tsp dried thyme
2.5ml/½ tsp dried chilli flakes
5ml/1 tsp vegetable bouillon powder
1 red pepper, seeded and diced
1 yellow pepper, seeded and diced
675g/1½lb/5¼ cups butternut squash or
    pumpkin, seeded and diced
salt and freshly ground black pepper
sprigs of thyme, to garnish

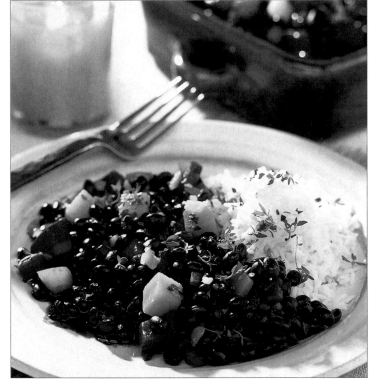

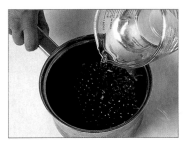

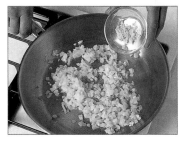

4 Add the peppers and squash or pumpkin, and mix well. Cover, then bake for 45 minutes until the vegetables are tender. Serve garnished with sprigs of thyme.

1 Soak the black beans overnight in plenty of water, then drain and rinse well. Place in a large saucepan, cover with fresh water and add the bay leaf. Bring to the boil, then boil rapidly for 10 minutes. Reduce the heat, cover and simmer for 30 minutes until tender. Drain, reserving the cooking water. Preheat the oven to 180°C/350°F/Gas 4.

2 Heat the oil and sauté the onion and garlic until softened. Add the mustard, molasses, sugar, thyme and chilli and cook for 1 minute. Stir in the black beans and spoon into a casserole.

3 Dilute the reserved cooking water to make 400ml/14fl oz/1⅔ cups. Mix in the bouillon powder and add to the casserole. Bake for 25 minutes.

NUTRITION NOTES	
Per portion:	
Energy	295Kcals/1234kJ
Fat, total	0.8g
saturated fat	0g
Protein	15.1g
Carbohydrate	61.4g
sugar, total	26.1g
Fibre – NSP	10.7g
Sodium	197mg

Pasta with Tomato and Chilli Sauce

Serve this simple dish with a green salad simply dressed in a little olive oil and lemon juice.

INGREDIENTS

Serves 4

450g/1lb passata
2 garlic cloves, crushed
150ml/¼ pint/⅔ cup dry white wine
15ml/1 tbsp sun-dried tomato purée
1 fresh red chilli
350g/12oz penne or other pasta shapes
15g/½oz/¼ cup finely chopped fresh flat leaf parsley
salt and freshly ground black pepper
freshly grated Pecorino cheese, to serve

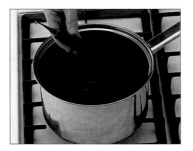

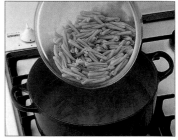

1 Put the passata, crushed garlic cloves, wine, sun-dried tomato purée and whole chilli in a saucepan and bring to the boil. Cover and simmer gently.

2 Cook the pasta in a large pan of boiling salted water for 10–12 minutes or until *al dente*.

3 Remove the chilli from the sauce and add half the parsley. Taste for seasoning. If you prefer a hotter taste, chop the chilli and add it to the sauce.

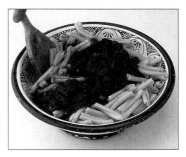

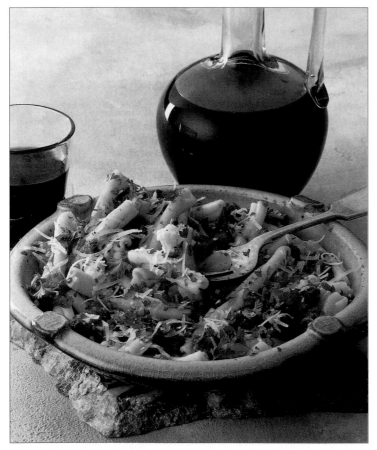

4 Drain the pasta and tip into a large, warmed bowl. Pour the sauce over the pasta and toss to mix. Serve at once, sprinkled with the grated Pecorino cheese and the remaining chopped fresh flat leaf parsley.

— NUTRITION NOTES —	
Per portion:	
Energy	350Kcals/1464kJ
Fat, total	1.7g
saturated fat	0.3g
Protein	11.8g
Carbohydrate	70.5g
sugar, total	5.8g
Fibre – NSP	3.6g
Sodium	64mg

Vegetable Medley

When tossed with freshly cooked pasta, this vegetable medley is ideal for a light lunch or supper. Allow about 450g/1lb dried pasta for this amount of sauce.

INGREDIENTS

Serves 4
2 carrots
1 courgette
75g/3oz French beans
1 small leek
5 plum tomatoes
handful of fresh flat leaf parsley
25g/1oz/2 tbsp butter
45ml/3 tbsp extra virgin olive oil
2.5ml/½ tsp granulated sugar
115g/4oz/1 cup frozen peas
salt and freshly ground black pepper

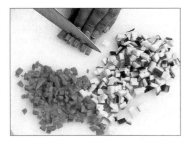

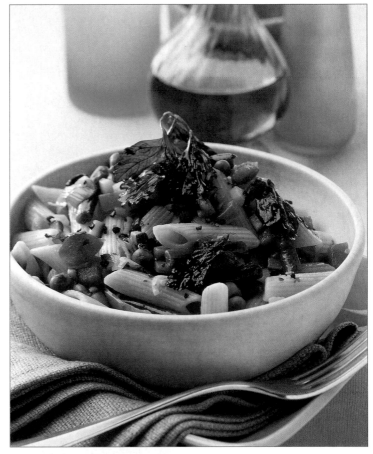

1 Dice the carrots and courgette finely. Top and tail the French beans, then cut them into 2cm/¾in lengths. Slice the leek thinly. Skin and dice the 5 tomatoes. Chop the flat leaf parsley and set aside.

2 Melt the butter in the oil in a medium frying pan or saucepan. When the mixture sizzles, add the prepared leek and carrots. Sprinkle the sugar over and fry, stirring frequently, for about 5 minutes.

3 Stir in the courgette, French beans and peas and season with plenty of salt and pepper. Cover and cook over a low to medium heat for 5–8 minutes until the vegetables are tender, stirring occasionally.

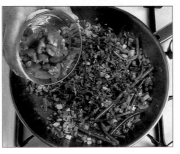

4 Stir in the parsley and chopped plum tomatoes and adjust the seasoning to taste. Serve at once, tossed with freshly cooked pasta.

— NUTRITION NOTES —	
Per portion:	
Energy	161Kcals/673kJ
Fat, total	14g
saturated fat	4.8g
Protein	2.9g
Carbohydrate	6.1g
sugar, total	3.7g
Fibre – NSP	3.2g
Sodium	60.4mg

Broccoli, Chilli and Artichoke Pasta

Chilli flakes add a fiery touch to this simple dish, proving that healthy eating can be exciting.

INGREDIENTS

Serves 6

350g/12oz/3 cups dried gnocchi pasta
300g/11oz broccoli florets
90ml/6 tbsp olive oil
1 large garlic clove, crushed
2.5–5ml/½–1 tsp dried chilli flakes
185g/6½oz/1½ cups artichoke hearts in oil, drained
salt and freshly ground black pepper
15ml/1 tbsp chopped fresh flat leaf parsley and grated Pecorino cheese, to garnish

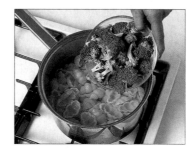

1 Cook the pasta in a large saucepan of boiling salted water according to the instructions on the packet until it is *al dente*. Add the broccoli for the last 3 minutes cooking time. Drain, reserving a little of the cooking water.

2 Meanwhile, heat the oil in a saucepan and sauté the garlic and chilli flakes for 1 minute. Add the pasta and vegetables and heat for 2 minutes. Add reserved water if necessary. Season and sprinkle with parsley and cheese.

NUTRITION NOTES	
Per portion:	
Energy	323Kcals/1351kJ
Fat, total	12.5g
saturated fat	1.8g
Protein	10.1g
Carbohydrate	45.9g
sugar, total	2.4g
Fibre – NSP	3.1g
Sodium	15mg

Buckwheat Pasta Bake

This bake is a spicy combination of nut-flavoured buckwheat pasta, vegetables and melted Fontina cheese.

INGREDIENTS

Serves 6

2 potatoes, cubed
225g/8oz/2 cups buckwheat pasta shapes, such as spirals
275g/10oz Savoy cabbage, shredded
45ml/3 tbsp olive oil, plus extra for greasing
1 onion, chopped
2 leeks, sliced
2 garlic cloves, chopped
175g/6oz brown cap mushrooms, thinly sliced
5ml/1 tsp caraway seeds
5ml/1 tsp cumin seeds
150ml/¼ pint/⅔ cup vegetable stock
150g/5oz/1¼ cups diced Fontina cheese
25g/1oz/¼ cup walnuts, roughly chopped (optional)
salt and freshly ground black pepper

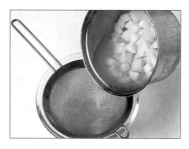

1 Preheat the oven to 200°C/400°F/ Gas 6. Oil a baking dish. Cook the potatoes in boiling salted water for 8–10 minutes, drain and set aside.

2 Cook the pasta and cabbage in boiling salted water for 2 minutes or until they are just cooked. Drain and rinse under cold running water.

3 Heat the oil in a large, heavy-based pan and fry the onion and leeks for 5 minutes until softened. Add the garlic and mushrooms and cook for a further 3 minutes, stirring occasionally, Stir in the spices and cook for 1 minute.

4 Add the cooked potatoes, pasta and cabbage and stir to combine, then season well. Spoon the mixture into the baking dish. Pour the stock over the vegetables, then sprinkle with the cheese and walnuts. Bake for about 15 minutes or until the cheese is melted and bubbling.

NUTRITION NOTES	
Per portion:	
Energy	359Kcals/1502kJ
Fat, total	17.9g
saturated fat	6.5g
Protein	13.1g
Carbohydrate	38.8g
sugar, total	5.3g
Fibre – NSP	4.4g
Sodium	482mg

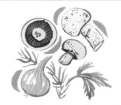

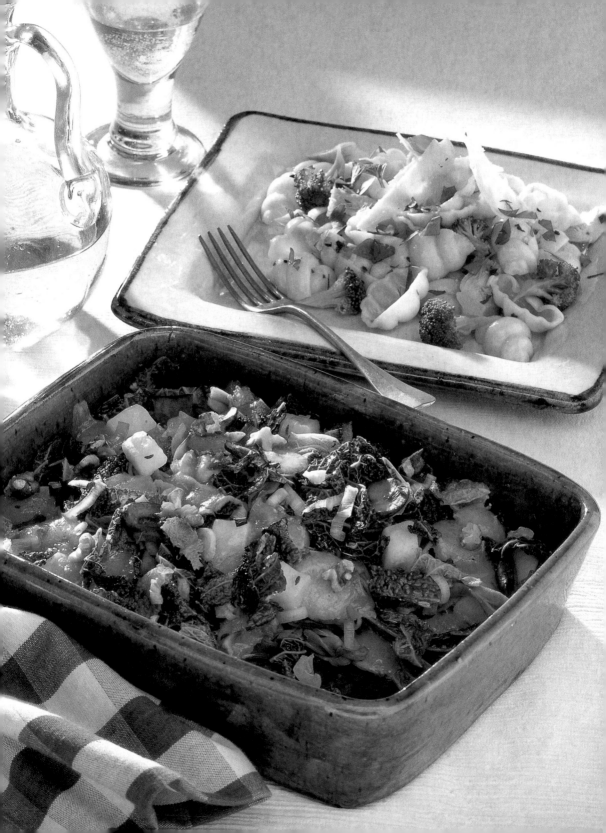

Polenta Pan-pizza

This yeast-free pizza is cooked in a frying pan rather than the oven. Serve with a simple tomato salad.

INGREDIENTS

Serves 4

30ml/2 tbsp olive oil
1 large red onion, sliced
3 garlic cloves, crushed
115g/4oz brown cap mushrooms, thinly sliced
5ml/1 tsp dried oregano
115g/4oz mozzarella cheese, crumbled
15ml/1 tbsp pine nuts (optional)

For the pizza base

50g/2oz/½ cup unbleached plain flour, sifted
2.5ml/½ tsp salt
115g/4oz/1 cup fine polenta
5ml/1 tsp baking powder
1 egg, beaten
150ml/¼ pint/⅔ cup milk
25g/1oz/⅓ cup Parmesan cheese freshly grated
2.5ml/½ tsp dried chilli flakes
15ml/1 tbsp olive oil

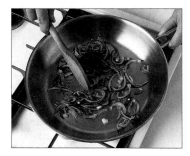

1 To make the topping, heat half the olive oil in a frying pan, add the onion and fry for 10 minutes until tender, stirring occasionally, Remove the onion from the pan and set aside.

2 Add the remaining oil to the pan and fry the garlic for 1 minute until slightly coloured, Add the mushrooms and oregano and cook for 5 minutes more until the mushrooms are tender.

3 To make the pizza base, mix together the flour, salt, polenta and baking powder in a bowl. Make a well in the centre and add the egg.

4 Gradually add the milk, and mix well with a fork to make into a thick, smooth batter. Stir in the Parmesan and chilli flakes.

5 Heat the olive oil in a 25cm/10in flameproof frying pan until very hot. Spoon in the batter and spread evenly. Cook over a moderate heat for about 3 minutes. Remove the pan from the heat and run a knife around the edge of the pizza base.

6 Place a plate over the pan and, holding them tightly together, flip over. Slide the pizza base back into the pan on its uncooked side and cook for 2 minutes until golden.

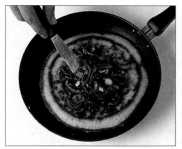

7 Preheat the grill to high. Spoon the onions over the base, then top with the mushroom mixture. Scatter the mozzarella on top, then grill for about 6 minutes until the mozzarella has melted. Sprinkle over the pine nuts (if using) and grill until golden. Serve cut into wedges.

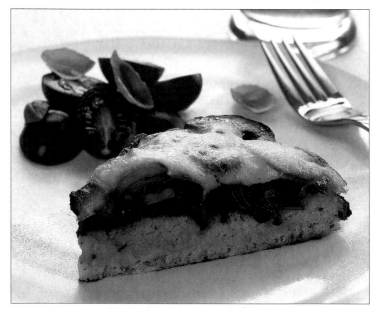

NUTRITION NOTES	
Per portion:	
Energy	386Kcals/1617kJ
Fat, total	19.3g
saturated fat	7g
Protein	16.5g
Carbohydrate	36.7g
sugar, total	4.1g
Fibre – NSP	1.25g
Sodium	685mg

Ricotta and Fontina Pizza

Pizza toppings can be very fattening but this is a light option incorporating garlic, mushrooms and fresh oregano.

INGREDIENTS

Serves 8

For the pizza dough
2.5ml/½ tsp active dried yeast
pinch of granulated sugar
450g/1lb/4 cups strong white flour
5ml/1 tsp salt
30ml/2 tbsp olive oil

For the tomato sauce
400g/14oz can chopped tomatoes
150ml/¼ pint/⅔ cup passata
1 large garlic clove, finely chopped
5ml/1 tsp dried oregano
1 bay leaf
10ml/2 tsp malt vinegar
salt and freshly ground black pepper

For the topping
30ml/2 tbsp olive oil, plus extra for
    brushing
1 garlic clove, finely chopped
350g/12oz mixed mushrooms
    (chestnut, flat or button), sliced
30ml/2 tbsp chopped fresh oregano,
    plus whole leaves, to garnish
250g/9oz/generous 1 cup ricotta
    cheese
225g/8oz Fontina cheese, sliced

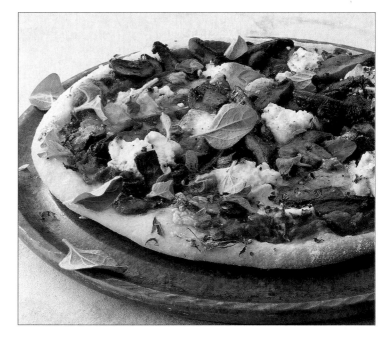

1 Make the dough. Put 300ml/½ pint/1 ¼ cups warm water in a measuring jug. Add the yeast and sugar and leave for 5–10 minutes until frothy. Sift the flour and salt into a large bowl and make a well in the centre. Gradually pour in the yeast mixture and the olive oil. Mix to make a smooth dough.

2 Transfer to a lightly floured surface and gently knead for about 10 minutes until smooth, springy and elastic. Place the dough in a floured bowl, cover and leave to rise in a warm place for about 1½ hours.

3 Meanwhile, make the tomato sauce. Place all the ingredients in a saucepan, cover and bring to the boil. Lower the heat, remove the lid and simmer for 20 minutes, stirring occasionally, until reduced.

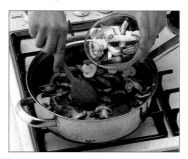

4 To make the topping, heat the oil in a frying pan and add the garlic and mushrooms, with salt and pepper to taste. Cook, stirring, for about 5 minutes or until the mushrooms are tender and golden. Set aside. Preheat the oven to 220°C/425°F/Gas 7.

5 Brush four baking sheets with oil. Knead the dough for 2 minutes, then divide into four equal pieces. Roll out each piece to a 25cm/10in round and place on a baking sheet.

6 Spoon the tomato sauce over each dough round. Brush the edges with a little olive oil. Add the mushrooms, chopped oregano and cheese. Bake for about 15 minutes until golden brown and crisp. Scatter the oregano leaves over just before serving.

NUTRITION NOTES	
Per pizza:	
Energy	408Kcals/1707kJ
Fat, total	19.2g
saturated fat	8.5g
Protein	16.4g
Carbohydrate	45.2g
sugar, total	3.4g
Fibre – NSP	2.7g
Sodium	531mg

Tomato and Pepper Rice

Tomato, pepper and fresh coriander taste delicious together in this light and colourful dish.

INGREDIENTS

Serves 4
30ml/2 tbsp sunflower oil
2.5ml/½ tsp onion seeds
1 onion, sliced
2 tomatoes, chopped
1 orange or yellow pepper, seeded
  and sliced
5ml/1 tsp crushed fresh root ginger
1 garlic clove, crushed
5ml/1 tsp chilli powder
1 potato, diced
7.5ml/1½ tsp salt
400g/14oz/2 cups basmati rice, soaked
750ml/1¼ pints/3 cups water
30–45ml/2–3 tbsp chopped coriander

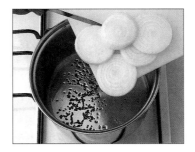

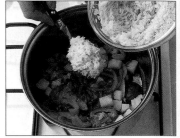

1 Heat the sunflower oil and fry the onion seeds for about 30 seconds. Add the sliced onion and fry for about 5 minutes until softened.

2 Stir in the tomatoes, pepper, ginger, garlic, chilli powder, potato and salt. Stir-fry over a medium heat for about 5 minutes more.

3 Drain the rice and add to the pan, then stir for about 1 minute until the grains are well coated.

4 Pour in the water and bring the rice to the boil, then lower the heat, cover the pan and cook the rice for 12–15 minutes. Remove from the heat, without lifting the lid, and leave the rice to stand for 5 minutes. Stir in the chopped coriander and serve.

COOK'S TIP

If you don't have any fresh tomatoes to hand you can use drained canned tomatoes.

NUTRITION NOTES

Per portion:

Energy	468Kcals/1958kJ
Fat, total	6.4g
saturated fat	0.8g
Protein	9.2g
Carbohydrate	92.7g
sugar, total	6.4g
Fibre – NSP	1.9g
Sodium	796mg

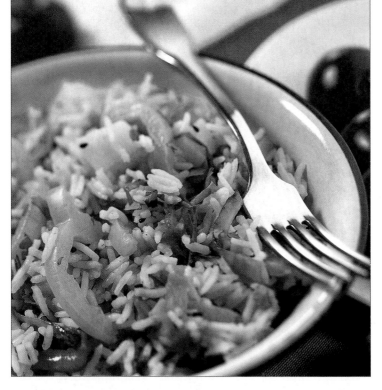

Vegetable Couscous

The combination of flavours ranges from the earthiness of onion to sweet, fruity prunes.

INGREDIENTS

Serves 4

15ml/3 tbsp olive oil
1 onion, chopped
2 garlic cloves, crushed
5ml/1 tsp ground cumin
5ml/1 tsp paprika
400g/14oz can chopped tomatoes
300ml/½ pint/1¼ cups vegetable stock
1 cinnamon stick
generous pinch of saffron strands
4 baby aubergines, quartered
8 baby courgettes, quartered
8 baby carrots
225g/8oz/1⅓ cups couscous
425g/15oz can chick peas, drained
175g/6oz/¾ cup prunes
45ml/3 tbsp chopped fresh parsley
45ml/3 tbsp chopped fresh coriander
10–15ml/2–3 tsp harissa sauce
salt

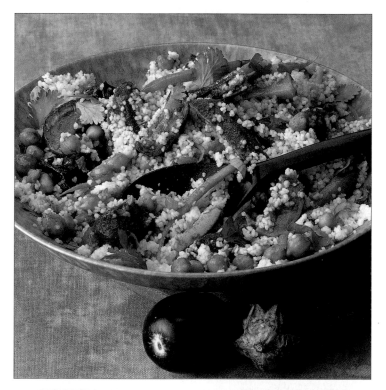

1 Heat the olive oil in a large saucepan. Add the onions and garlic and cook gently for 5 minutes until soft. Add the cumin and paprika and cook, stirring, for 1 minute.

2 Add the tomatoes, vegetable stock, cinnamon stick, saffron, aubergines, courgettes and carrots. Season with salt. Bring to the boil, cover, lower the heat and cook for 20 minutes until the vegetables are just tender.

NUTRITION NOTES	
Per portion:	
Energy	474Kcals/1983kJ
Fat, total	13.3g
saturated fat	1.7g
Protein	17.1g
Carbohydrate	75.9g
sugar, total	28.7g
Fibre – NSP	12.3g
Sodium	485mg

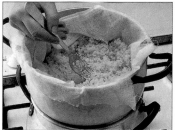

3 Line a steamer, metal sieve or colander with a double thickness of muslin. Soak the couscous according to the instructions on the packet. Add the chick peas and prunes to the vegetables and cook for 5 minutes. Fork the couscous to break up any lumps and then spread it in the prepared steamer. Place on top of the vegetables, cover, and gently cook for 5 minutes until the couscous is hot.

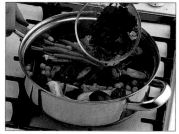

4 Stir the parsley and coriander into the vegetables. Heap the couscous on to a warmed serving plate. Using a slotted spoon, arrange the vegetables on top. Spoon over a little sauce and toss gently to combine. Stir the harissa into the remaining sauce and serve separately.

PROPERTY OF
WALNUT PUBLIC
LIBRARY DISTRICT

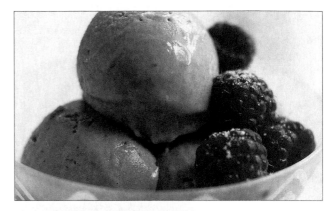

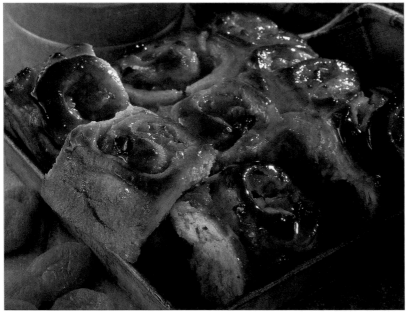

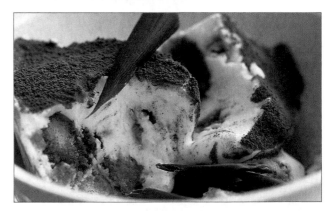

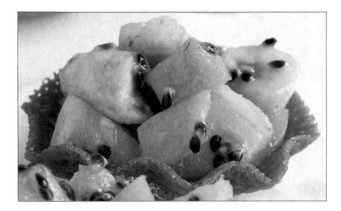

DESSERTS

The dessert is the crowning glory of a meal and, for many people,

their all-time favourite course. Go easy on the sugar and let

fruit give its natural sweetness to your desserts. If you also select

low-fat dairy products, such as fromage frais and yogurt,

your puddings will be both healthy and nutritious and not the lapses

in dietary principles that people tend to associate with dessert. There's

enough choice here to suit all palates.

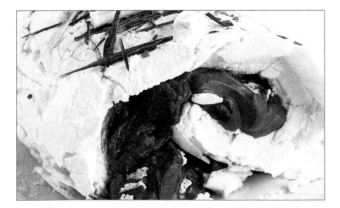

Spiced Fruit Compote

This delicately spiced fruit compote is ideal for the winter months when fresh fruit is sometimes limited. Serve with pancakes, frozen yogurt or fat-free sponge cake as a dessert, or with natural yogurt for breakfast.

INGREDIENTS

Serves 4

250g/9oz mixed dried fruits, such as apples, apricots, pears and prunes
1 cinnamon stick
3 whole green cardamom pods, lightly crushed
400ml/14fl oz/1⅔ cups apple and mango juice
5ml/1 tsp cornflour

1 Place the mixed dried fruit, cinnamon and cardamom in a large bowl. Pour over the juice and 400ml/14fl oz/1⅔ cups of boiling water. Allow to cool, cover and leave overnight in the fridge.

NUTRITION NOTES	
Per portion:	
Energy	205Kcals/857kJ
Fat, total	0.3g
saturated fat	0g
Protein	1.5g
Carbohydrate	52.4g
sugar, total	52.4g
Fibre – NSP	1.4g
Sodium	32mg

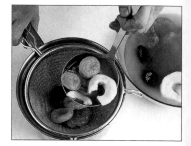

2 Remove the cardamom pods and cinnamon from the fruit. Mix the cornflour with cold water to make a smooth paste. Drain the liquid from the fruit into a small saucepan. Stir in the cornflour and bring to the boil; cook for1 minute,stirring. Cool and return to the fruit.

Warm Tropical Fruit Salad Baskets

Baking fruit seems to enhance its sweetness and fruity flavour, and makes a pleasant change from fresh fruit salad.

INGREDIENTS

Serves 4

1 ripe pineapple, peeled and cubed
2 large ripe mangoes, skinned, stoned and cubed
2 bananas, peeled and thickly sliced
4 passion fruit, seeded
60ml/4 tbsp demerara sugar
25g/1oz/2 tbsp unsalted butter
zest and juice of 1 large orange
4 brandy snaps
fresh mint, to decorate

COOK'S TIP
This recipe is ideally suited for you to use whatever seasonal fruit is to hand – try star fruit, papaya and watermelon.

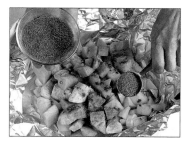

1 Preheat the oven to 200°C/400°F/ Gas 6. Place the fruit on a large foil square, draw together the edges to make a parcel, but before you close it, add the sugar, butter and orange juice and zest. Bake for 15 minutes.

2 Place the brandy snaps on a baking tray in the oven for 1 minute. Remove from the oven and unroll them so they become flat. Place over an orange or an upturned tumbler and shape into a basket. Allow to set.

3 Remove the fruit from the foil and spoon into the brandy snap baskets. Decorate with a little fresh mint and serve immediately.

NUTRITION NOTES	
Per portion:	
Energy	299Kcals/1251kJ
Fat, total	8.6g
saturated fat	3.5g
Protein	2.2g
Carbohydrate	56.6g
sugar, total	52.5g
Fibre – NSP	3.7g
Sodium	90.2mg

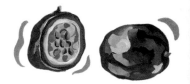

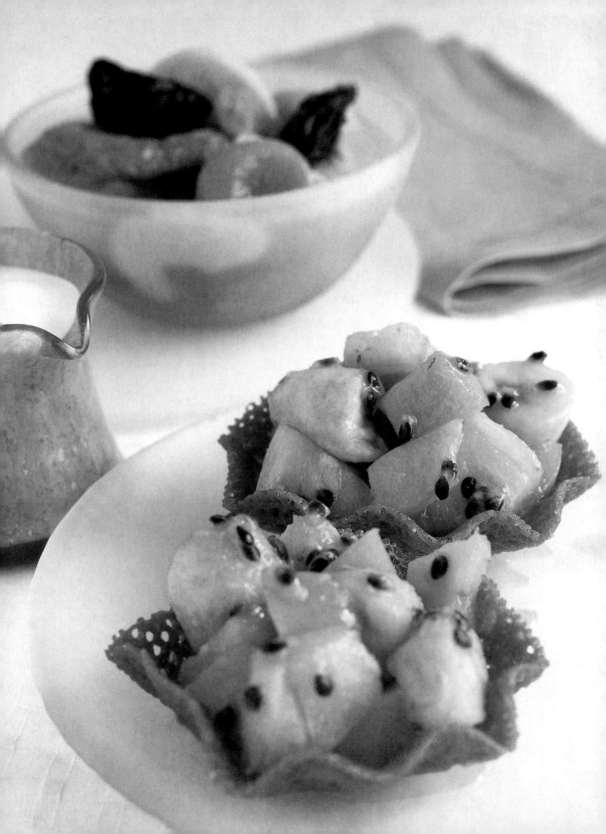

Raspberry Sherbet

This modern adaption of the classic sherbet is made from raspberry purée blended with sugar syrup and virtually fat-free fromage frais, rather than milk.

INGREDIENTS

Serves 6

175g/6oz/¾ cup caster sugar
150ml/¼ pint/⅔ cup water
500g/1¼lb/3⅓ cups raspberries, plus
   extra to serve
500ml/17fl oz/generous 2 cups
   virtually fat-free fromage frais

COOK'S TIP

If you are using an ice cream maker, check your handbook: this recipe makes 900ml/1½ pints/3¾ cups of mixture; if this is too much for your machine, make it in two batches.

---

1 Put the sugar and water in a small saucepan and bring to the boil, stirring until the sugar has dissolved. Pour into a jug and cool.

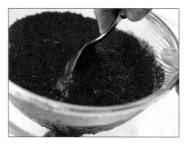

2 Put 350g/12oz/2⅓ cups of the raspberries in a food processor or blender. Process to a purée, then, using the back of a spoon, press through a sieve placed over a large bowl to remove the seeds. Stir the sugar syrup into the raspberry purée and chill the mixture until it is very cold.

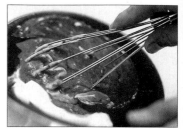

3 Add the fromage frais to the chilled purée and whisk until smooth. If you are using an ice cream maker, churn for 25–30 minutes until thick. If you are making it by hand, pour the mixture into a freezerproof container and freeze for 4 hours, beating once with a fork, electric whisk or in a food processor to break up the ice crystals.

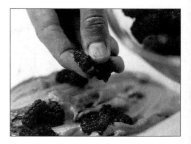

4 Scrape the sherbet into a plastic tub and beat it again. Crush the remaining raspberries and add them to the sherbet. Mix lightly, freeze for 2–3 hours until firm. Scoop into dishes and serve with extra raspberries.

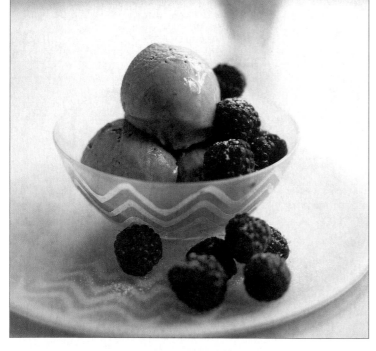

NUTRITION NOTES

Per portion:

Energy	184Kcals/769kJ
Fat, total	0.4g
saturated fat	0.2g
Protein	7.6g
Carbohydrate	40.1g
sugar, total	40.1g
Fibre – NSP	2.1g
Sodium	31.5mg

Iced Tiramisu

This favourite Italian dessert makes a marvellous ice cream. It tastes very rich, despite its virtually fat-free content.

INGREDIENTS

Serves 6

150g/5oz/¾ cup caster sugar
150ml/¼ pint/⅔ cup water
250g/9oz/generous 1 cup mascarpone cheese
200g/7oz/scant 1 cup virtually fat-free fromage frais
5ml/1 tsp vanilla essence
10ml/2 tsp instant coffee, dissolved in 30ml/2 tbsp boiling water
30ml/2 tbsp coffee liqueur or brandy
75g/3oz sponge finger biscuits
cocoa powder, for dusting
chocolate curls, to decorate

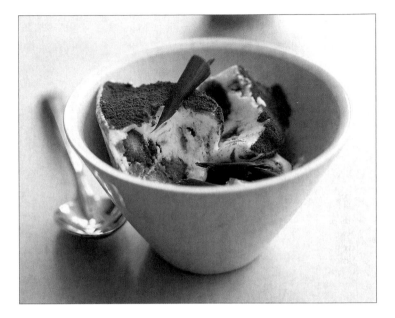

1 Put 115g/4oz/½ cup of the sugar into a small saucepan. Add the water and bring to the boil, stirring until the sugar has dissolved. Let the syrup cool, then chill it.

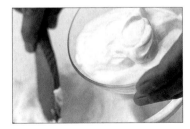

2 Put the mascarpone into a bowl. Beat it with a spoon until it is soft, then stir in the fromage frais. Add the chilled sugar syrup, a little at a time, then stir in the vanilla essence.

COOK'S TIP

Do allow time for the ice cream to soften in the fridge before scooping it, especially if it was made the day before, because home-made ice creams freeze much harder than commercial ones.

3 If using an ice cream maker, churn the mascarpone mixture until it is thick but too soft to scoop. If you are making the ice cream by hand, spoon the mixture into a plastic tub or similar freezerproof container and freeze for 4 hours, beating once with a fork to break up the ice crystals.

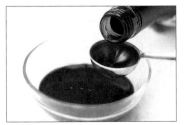

4 Meanwhile, put the coffee mixture in a small bowl, sweeten with the remaining sugar, then add the liqueur or brandy. Stir and leave to cool.

5 Crumble the biscuits into small pieces and toss them in the coffee mixture. If you have frozen the ice cream in a tub, beat it again.

6 Whichever way you've made the ice cream, spoon a third of it into a 900ml/1½ pint/4 cup plastic container, or other freezerproof container. Spoon over half the biscuits, then top with half the remaining ice cream.

7 Sprinkle the last of the coffee-soaked biscuits over the top and cover with the remaining ice cream. Freeze for 2–3 hours until firm and able to be scooped. Dust with cocoa powder and spoon into glass dishes. Decorate with chocolate curls.

NUTRITION NOTES

Per portion:

Energy	384Kcals/1606kJ
Fat, total	5.5g
saturated fat	2.9g
Protein	11.5g
Carbohydrate	61g
sugar, total	38.7g
Fibre – NSP	0.13g
Sodium	80mg

Pan-fried Apple Slices with Walnut Shortbread

Soft, caramelized apples and crisp, nutty shortbread make a perfect combination. Serve warm with a spoonful of low-fat yogurt or virtually fat-free fromage frais.

INGREDIENTS

Serves 6

25g/1oz/2 tbsp unsalted butter
4 dessert apples, cored and thinly sliced
30ml/2 tbsp soft light brown sugar
10ml/2 tsp ground ginger
5ml/1 tsp ground cinnamon
2.5ml/½ tsp grated nutmeg

For the walnut shortbread

75g/3oz/⅔ cup wholemeal flour
75g/3oz/⅔ cup unbleached plain flour
25g/1oz/¼ cup oatmeal
5ml/1 tsp baking powder
1.5ml/¼ tsp salt
50g/2oz/¼ cup golden caster sugar
115g/4oz/8 tbsp unsalted butter
40g/1½oz/¼ cup walnuts,
    finely chopped
15ml/1 tbsp milk, plus extra
    for brushing
demerera sugar, for sprinkling

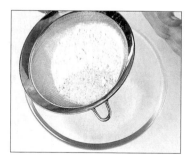

1 Preheat the oven to 180°C/350°F/ Gas 4 and grease one or two baking sheets. To make the walnut shortbread, sift together the two flours, adding any bran left in the sieve, and mix with the oatmeal, baking powder, salt and sugar. Rub in the butter with your fingers until the mixture resembles fine breadcrumbs.

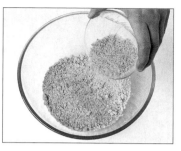

2 Add the chopped walnuts to the mixture, then stir in enough of the milk to form a soft dough.

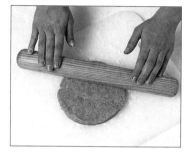

3 Gently knead the dough on a floured work surface. Form into a round, then roll out to a 5mm/¼in thickness. Using a 5cm/2½in fluted cutter, stamp out twelve rounds – you may have some dough left over.

NUTRITION NOTES	
Per portion:	
Energy	398Kcals/1664kJ
Fat, total	24.4g
saturated fat	13.2g
Protein	4.6g
Carbohydrate	42.5g
sugar, total	22g
Fibre – NSP	3.2g
Sodium	181mg

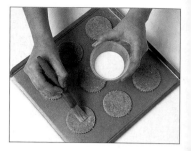

4 Place the shortbread rounds on the prepared baking sheets. Brush the tops with milk and sprinkle with sugar. Bake for 12–15 minutes until golden brown, then transfer to a wire rack and leave to cool.

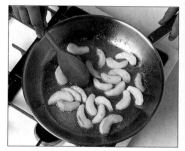

5 To prepare the apples, melt the butter in a heavy-based frying pan. Add the apples and cook for 3–4 minutes over a gentle heat until softened. Increase the heat to medium, add the sugar and spices, and stir well. Cook for a few minutes, stirring frequently, until the sauce turns golden brown and caramelizes.

6 Place two shortbread rounds on each of four individual serving plates and spoon over the warm apples and sauce. Serve immediately.

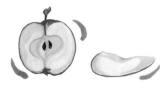

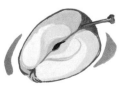

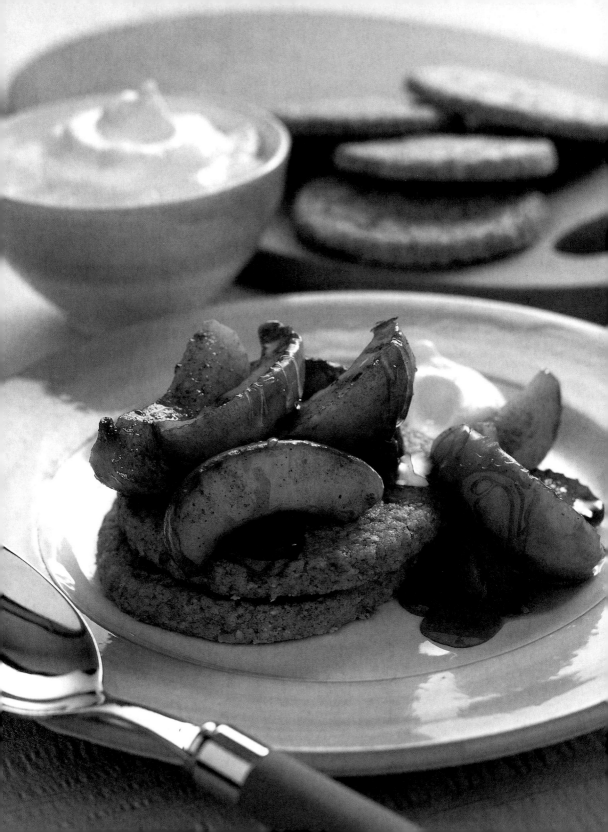

Spiced Apple Cake

Grated apple and chopped dates
give this cake a natural sweetness.

INGREDIENTS

Serves 8

225g/8oz/2 cups self-raising
   wholemeal flour
5ml/1 tsp baking powder
10ml/2 tsp ground cinnamon
175g/6oz/1 cup chopped dates
75g/3oz/⅓ cup light muscovado sugar
15ml/1 tbsp pear and apple spread
120ml/4fl oz/½ cup apple juice
2 eggs
90ml/6 tbsp sunflower oil
2 eating apples, cored and grated
15ml/1 tbsp chopped walnuts

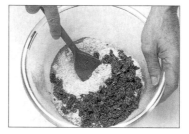

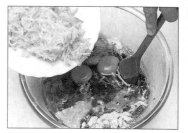

1 Preheat the oven to 180°C/350°F/
Gas 4. Grease and line a deep,
round 20cm/8in cake tin. Sift the flour,
baking powder and cinnamon into a
mixing bowl, then add the dates and
mix into the dry ingredients. Make a
well in the centre.

2 Mix the sugar with the pear and
apple spread in a small bowl.
Gradually stir in the apple juice. Add to
the dry ingredients with the eggs, oil
and apples. Mix thoroughly.

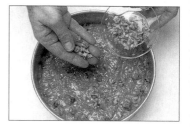

3 Spoon the mixture into the cake
tin, sprinkle with the walnuts and
bake for 60 minutes or until a skewer
inserted into the cake's centre comes
out clean. Transfer to a rack, remove
the lining paper and leave to cool.

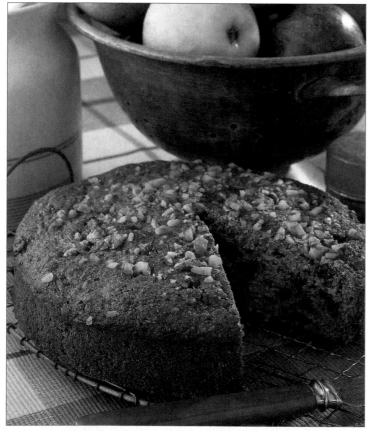

NUTRITION NOTES

Per portion:

Energy	313Kcals/1309kJ
Fat, total	11.7g
saturated fat	1.6g
Protein	6.5g
Carbohydrate	48.4g
sugar, total	31g
Fibre – NSP	3.9g
Sodium	25mg

COOK'S TIP

Leave the apple peel on – the skin adds
extra fibre and softens on cooking.

Chocolate Roulade

Even when you're watching your weight, you still need to indulge yourself every now and then.

INGREDIENTS

Serves 6

4 egg whites
225g/8oz/1 cup caster sugar
15ml/1 tbsp cornflour
15ml/1 tbsp malt vinegar
5ml/1 tsp vanilla essence
125g/4oz chocolate and hazelnut
    spread
200ml/7fl oz/1 cup Greek yogurt
icing sugar, for dusting
chocolate shavings, to decorate

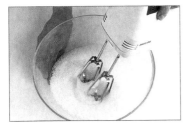

1 Preheat the oven to 150°C/300°F/ Gas 2. Line the base and sides of a 31.5 x 21.5cm/12½ x 8½in Swiss roll tin with baking parchment. With an electric whisk, beat the egg whites until frothy and doubled in bulk, then whisk in the sugar until the mixture is very thick and shiny. Whisk in the cornflour, vinegar and vanilla essence.

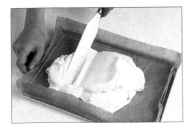

2 Spoon the mixture into the prepared tin and level the surface. Bake in the oven for 50 minutes or until just firm on the surface.

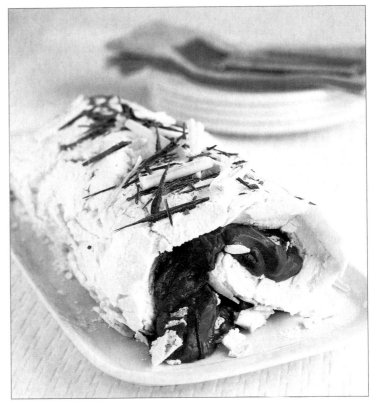

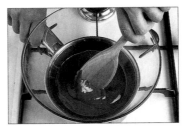

3 Place the chocolate spread in a bowl over boiling water and heat, stirring, until soft. Place the yogurt in a bowl and stir in the melting chocolate.

4 Dust a sheet of baking parchment with icing sugar. Allow the meringue to cool for 10 minutes, then turn out on to the baking parchment and carefully peel off the paper.

5 Spread the yogurt mixture over the meringue and then, using the paper to help you, roll from one of the long ends as you would a Swiss roll. Chill for 30 minutes. Dust with a little more icing sugar and decorate with chocolate curls.

NUTRITION NOTES	
Per portion:	
Energy	316Kcals/1322kJ
Fat, total	9.9g
saturated fat	3.8g
Protein	5.4g
Carbohydrate	54.9g
sugar, total	52.4g
Fibre – NSP	0.2g
Sodium	77.7mg

Banana and Apricot Chelsea Buns

Old favourites are given a low-fat twist with a delectable banana and apricot fruit filling.

INGREDIENTS

Serves 9
90ml/6 tbsp warm skimmed milk
5ml/1 tsp dried yeast
pinch of sugar
225g/8oz/2 cups strong plain flour
10ml/2 tsp mixed spice
2.5ml/½ tsp salt
25g/1oz/2 tbsp soft margarine
50g/2oz/¼ cup caster sugar
1 egg

For the filling
1 large ripe banana
175g/6oz/¾ cup ready-to-eat dried
  apricots
30ml/2 tbsp light muscovado sugar

For the glaze
30ml/2 tbsp caster sugar
30ml/2 tbsp water

1 Grease an 18cm/7in square cake tin. Put the warm milk in a jug. Sprinkle the yeast on top. Add a pinch of sugar to help activate the yeast, mix well and leave for 30 minutes.

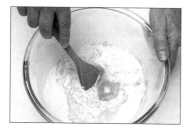

2 Sift the flour, spice and salt into a mixing bowl. Rub in the margarine, then stir in the sugar. Make a central well, pour in the yeast mixture and the egg. Gradually mix in the flour to make a soft dough, adding extra milk if needed.

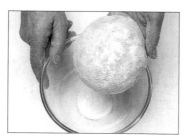

3 Turn the dough out on to a floured surface and knead for 5 minutes until smooth and elastic. Return to the clean bowl, cover with a damp dish towel and leave in a warm place to rise for 2 hours or until doubled in bulk.

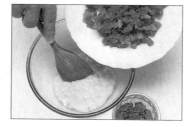

4 Meanwhile, prepare the filling. Mash the banana in a bowl. Using scissors, snip the apricots, then stir into the banana with the sugar.

COOK'S TIP

Do not leave the buns in the tin for too long or the glaze will stick to the sides, making them very difficult to remove.

NUTRITION NOTES

Per portion:

Energy	196Kcals/820kJ
Fat, total	3.5g
saturated fat	0.7g
Protein	4.9g
Carbohydrate	38.8g
sugar, total	20.1g
Fibre – NSP	2.2g
Sodium	37.3mg

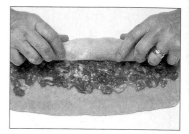

5 Knead the risen dough on a lightly floured surface for 2 minutes, then roll out to a 30 x 23cm/12 x 9in rectangle. Spread the banana and apricot filling over the dough and roll up lengthways like a Swiss roll, with the join underneath.

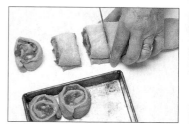

6 Cut the roll into 9 pieces and place, cut side down, in the prepared tin. Cover and leave to rise in a warm place for about 30 minutes. Preheat the oven to 200°C/400°F/Gas 6.

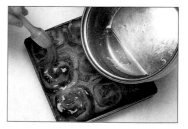

7 Bake the buns for 20–25 minutes. Meanwhile, make the glaze. Mix the sugar and water in a small saucepan. Heat, stirring, until dissolved, then boil for 2 minutes. Brush the glaze over the buns while still hot, then remove them from the tin and leave them to cool.

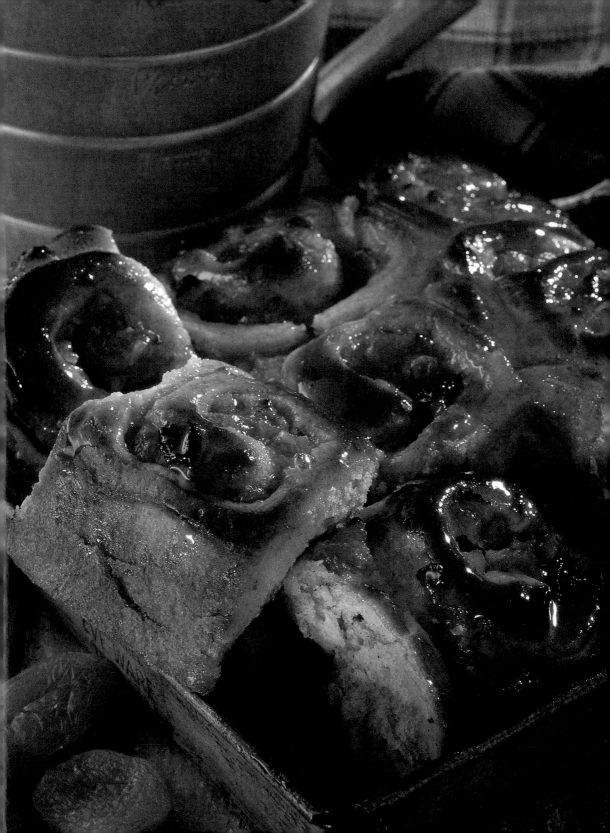

Index

apples: pan-fried apple slices with walnut
  shortbread, 90
  spiced apple cake, 92
apricots: banana and apricot chelsea buns, 94
artichokes: broccoli, chilli and artichoke
  pasta, 78

bacon, mushrooms with thyme, lemon
  and, 34
bananas: banana and apricot chelsea buns, 94
  banana and walnut muffins, 33
  banana smoothie, 28
beancurd: hot-and-sour soup, 40
beans, 16, 22
  black bean hotpot, 75
  cannellini bean and rosemary toasts, 42
  spinach and cannellini beans, 70
beansprouts: coriander omelette parcels, 43
beef: beef teriyaki, 56
  ravioli with Bolognese sauce, 57
biryani, chicken, 63
black bean hotpot, 75
Bolognese sauce, ravioli with, 57
bread, 22
  cannellini bean and rosemary toasts, 42
broccoli, chilli and artichoke pasta, 78
buckwheat pasta bake, 78

cake, spiced apple, 92
calories, 8–9, 11, 20–3, 24
cannellini beans: cannellini bean and
  rosemary toasts, 42
  spinach and cannellini beans, 70
carrot and courgette frittata, 35
ceviche, 45
cheese, 16, 19, 20
  iced tiramisu, 89
  ravioli with Bolognese sauce, 57
  ricotta and fontina pizza, 81
chelsea buns, banana and apricot, 94
chicken: chicken biryani, 63
  chicken in herb crusts, 62

chicken with cashew nuts, 60
  grilled chicken salad with lavender, 46
  pasta bows with chicken and cherry
  tomatoes, 61
chillies: pasta with tomato and chilli sauce, 76
chive and potato scones, 32
chocolate roulade, 93
clam and pasta soup, 38
cooking techniques, 18
coriander omelette parcels, 43
courgettes: carrot and courgette frittata, 35
couscous, vegetable, 83
cranberry juice: cool cranberry smoothie, 28
crash diets, 11
curried potatoes and spinach, 74

dairy products, 16, 20
dressings, 22

eggs, 15, 22
  carrot and courgette frittata, 35
  coriander omelette parcels, 43
exercise, 9

fad diets, 11
fat, 20–3
  in diet, 10, 17
  keeping to a minimum, 19
  storage in body, 6–7
frittata, carrot and courgette, 35
fruit, 14, 23
  spiced fruit compote, 86
  warm tropical fruit salad baskets, 86

garlic soup, 39
granola, 30

ham: stir-fried jewelled rice, 66
herb crusts, chicken in, 62
hot-and-sour soup, 40

kebabs: marinated lamb kebabs, 54
  monkfish and scallop skewers, 64
tropical fruit smoothie, 28

lamb: marinated lamb kebabs, 54
  spicy meatballs with red rice, 55
lavender, grilled chicken salad with, 46
limes: ceviche, 45
mangoes: totally tropical smoothie, 28
spicy meatballs with red rice, 55
monkfish and scallop skewers, 64
muesli, luxury, 30

muffins, banana and walnut, 33
mushrooms with bacon, thyme and
  lemon, 34

oats: granola, 30
  luxury muesli, 30
omelette parcels, coriander, 43

passion fruit: tropical fruit smoothie, 28
pasta: broccoli, chilli and artichoke pasta, 78
  buckwheat pasta bake, 78
  clam and pasta soup, 38
  pasta bows with chicken and cherry
  tomatoes, 61
  ravioli with Bolognese sauce, 57
  seafood conchiglie, 65
  vegetables and pasta salad, 50
  with tomato and chilli sauce, 76
pear: banana smoothie, 28
peppers: baked sweet potato salad, 49
  marinated lamb kebabs, 54
  tomato rice, 82
  yellow tomato and orange pepper salsa, 44
pineapple juice: totally tropical smoothie, 28
pizzas: polenta pan-pizza, 80
  ricotta and fontina pizza, 81
polenta pan-pizza, 80
pork, sweet-and-sour, 58
potatoes: chive and potato scones, 32
  curried potatoes and spinach, 74
  mixed vegetable and new potato
  casserole, 71
  potato and mixed vegetable salad, 51
prawns: ceviche, 45
prune purée, 19

raspberries: tropical fruit smoothie, 28
  raspberry sherbet, 88
ravioli with Bolognese sauce, 57
rice, 22
  chicken biryani, 63
  roasted vegetables with salsa verde, 72
  spicy meatballs with red rice, 55
  stir-fried jewelled rice, 66
  tomato rice, 82
ricotta and fontina pizza, 81
rocket: seafood salad, 65
roulade, chocolate, 93

salads: grilled chicken salad with lavender, 46
  potato and mixed vegetable salad, 51
  seafood conchiglie, 65
  baked sweet potato salad, 49
  vegetable and pasta salad, 50

salmon, ceviche, 45
salsas: roasted vegetables with salsa verde, 72
  yellow tomato and orange pepper salsa, 44
scallops: ceviche, 45
  monkfish and scallop skewers, 64
  seafood conchiglie, 65
scones, chive and potato, 32
sea bass en papillote, 67
seafood conchiglie, 65
sherbet, raspberry, 88
shortbread, walnut, 90
smoothies, 28
soups: clam and pasta soup, 38
  garlic soup, 39
  hot-and-sour soup, 40
spinach: curried potatoes and spinach, 74
  spinach and cannellini beans, 70
strawberries: cool cranberry smoothie, 28
sweet-and-sour pork, 58
sweet potato salad, baked, 49

tiramisu, iced, 89
toasts, cannellini bean and rosemary, 42
tomatoes: pasta bows with chicken and cherry
  tomatoes, 61
  pasta with tomato and chilli sauce, 76
  tomato and pepper rice, 82
  yellow tomato and orange pepper salsa, 44
totally tropical smoothie, 28
tuna carpaccio, 48

vegetables, 14, 23, 69–83
  buckwheat pasta bake, 78
  mixed vegetable and new potato
  casserole, 71
  roasted vegetables with salsa verde, 72
  vegetable couscous, 83
  vegetable medley, 77
  vegetables and pasta salad, 50

waist measurements, 7
walnuts: banana and walnut muffins, 33
  walnut shortbread, 90
water, drinking, 12